D1569816

BEHAVIOR DISORDERS
OF CHILDHOOD
AND ADOLESCENCE

BEHAVIOR DISORDERS
OF CHILDHOOD
AND ADOLESCENCE

By

RICHARD L. JENKINS, M.D.
Professor Emeritus of Child Psychiatry
University of Iowa College of Medicine
Iowa City, Iowa

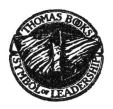

CHARLES C THOMAS · PUBLISHER
Springfield · Illinois · U.S.A.

Published and Distributed Throughout the World by
CHARLES C THOMAS • PUBLISHER
BANNERSTONE HOUSE
301-327 East Lawrence Avenue, Springfield, Illinois, U.S.A.

© *1973, by* CHARLES C THOMAS • PUBLISHER
ISBN 0-398-02786-2
Library of Congress Catalog Card Number: 72-93216

Printed in the United States of America
W-2

PREFACE

T HE SECOND EDITION of the Diagnostic and Statistical Manual of Mental Disorders of the American Psychiatric Association includes a new category—*behavior disorders of childhood and adolescence*—which is taken from the Eighth Revision of the International Classification of Diseases. "This major category is reserved for disorders occurring in childhood or adolescence that are more stable, internalized and resistent to treatment than *transient situational disturbances* but less so than *psychoses, neuroses* and *personality disorders.* This intermediate stability is attributed to the greater fluidity of all behavior at this age."

We should note that there has as yet been no adequate discussion of these behavior disorders organized around the subdivisions of the above-named diagnostic categories.

This book is written primarily for professional workers who deal with maladjusted and problem children—psychiatrists, pediatricians, family physicians, psychologists, social workers, teachers in special education, etc. It is an effort to provide a broad framework for the understanding of maladjusted children, and to assist in the task of readjustment and rehabilitation. While the analysis of the evidence has required some technical use of a computer, I have endeavored to state the results in non-technical language, understandable to all humanly perceptive readers.

Hopefully this small volume will help to clarify the reasons for some repetitive human behavior which is maladaptive in our society, and particularly to shed some light on methods available for reducing such maladaptive behavior and replacing it with behavior more adaptive and more appropriate.

Iowa City, Iowa   R.L.J.

CONTENTS

BEHAVIOR DISORDERS
OF CHILDHOOD
AND ADOLESCENCE

CHAPTER 1

THE NATURE OF THE PROBLEM

THE FORESTS GRADUALLY WITHERED AND DRIED UP. AS THE TREES LOST THEIR LEAVES AND DIED, OUR REMOTE ANCESTORS HAD TO SHIFT FROM THE TREES TO THE GROUND IN SEARCH OF FOOD. INASMUCH AS THE REMAINING FORESTS WERE OCCUPIED BY THEIR OWN ARBOREAL POPULATIONS, OUR ANCESTORS ADAPTED THEMSELVES GRADUALLY TO LIVING ON THE SAVANNAH, SPENDING MORE AND MORE TIME IN AN ERECT POSTURE. THIS FREED THEIR HANDS AND ARMS FROM THE HEAVY TASK OF LOCOMOTION, AND MADE IT POSSIBLE FOR THEM TO PICK UP AND USE STICKS AND STONES AS PRIMITIVE TOOLS OR WEAPONS. THE SURVIVAL OF THESE REMOTE ANCESTORS OF OURS DEPENDED UPON A BEHAVIORAL ADAPTATION OF THE FIRST MAGNITUDE.

Lacking claws or teeth effective for fighting, lacking speed in comparison with most quadrupeds, they had to evolve tools, weapons, and teamwork, and learn effectively to cooperate in their pursuit of a livelihood and in repulsing predators. Out of these changes was to emerge the most adaptive and adaptable of animals—MAN. Man is distinguished most of all by the extent to which learned behavior has replaced genetically determined inborn responses.

We see genetically determined inborn responses most highly developed in the insects and arachnids. Different species of spiders, for example, differ widely in the design and architecture of the webs they weave. No one teaches a spider to weave a web, and certainly no one has been able to teach a spider to weave a second kind of web. The pattern of web-making is a pre-formed, inherited, automatic response.

3

Inborn, Instinctual Responses

The human animal has a relative dearth of the well-defined, pre-formed automatic responses such as characterize the instinctive behavior of insects. The sucking reflex in the newborn is indeed of this specific and pre-formed character. But as we see "instinctual" elements in the behavior of adolescents and of adults, they appear as awakening areas of emotional responsiveness rather than as behavior manifestations of pre-formed patterns of response. Indeed they are subject to modification or blocking by many elements in the complexities of human life.

There is clearly a correlation between breast feeding and maternal acceptance, but the problem of causality in this relation takes on some of the character of the old question, "Which came first, the chicken or the egg?" That there is, in fact, a circular reinforcement seems highly probable.

The human maternal response is obviously a highly complex reaction influenced by instinct, habit, value systems, the satisfactoriness of the ongoing life adjustment, and the current significance of the offspring to the mother. That is to say, a socially secure mother in a happy marriage without economic hardship has a very different set of external pressures influencing (and reinforcing) her maternal responses than does the unmarried early-teenage mother of an illegitimate child. Some years ago when a five year old girl in Chile gave birth to a child and thereby made the medical annals, it was reported that she was interested in her dolls, but not in her baby. Something went wrong biologically and sexual maturity developed in early childhood, thereby grossly preceding the time of growing up emotionally. Surely it does not seem surprising that, at this age, the anlage of the maternal response had not developed further.

The newborn has only limited potentialities for interaction with the mother; only the most vital ones such as those of sucking and registering distress by crying are well-developed at birth. Out of repetitive ministrations to the infant's helplessness, the maternal response becomes a part of the mother. Initially almost all the flexibility and adaptiveness is necessarily on the maternal side, but a specificity of response to the mother begins to develop on the side of the infant. Early in the infant's development there is an amazing, if gradual recognition of the mother as another person, the differentiation of her from other adults and, under favorable circumstances, developing confidence, trust, and psychological dependence. Perhaps the most paradoxical element here is that it is the infant's experience of successful and fulfilled dependence that leads to the capacity for successful independence, exploration, and the adaptive and creative behavior of which the human animal is capable. This potential is compounded of a basic confidence, a secondarily developed and developing sense of self, of self-belief and self-confidence, an uninhibited curiosity in the seeking of new experience, and a zest for living. All of this depends upon a highly complicated and successful interaction principally between two different individuals, the mother and the developing infant.

Learned Responses in the Individuals

Man does show his kinship with the rest of the mammalian world in the dual nature of his behavioral controls. On the one hand, his behavior is under the control of the more recently evolved portions of his central nervous system, particularly his cerebral cortex, with its capacity to analyze a problem and find a solution. On the other hand, there are the more primitive controls of strong emotion—fear, anger, love—which touch autonomic responses more or less appropriate to a particular kind of situation and may be reinforced by chemical controllers (as nor-adrenalin or adrenalin) released into the blood stream. The result may be an emotional and physiological weighing of the balance in favor of a particular pattern of action, such as flight or fighting.

If we create the abstraction of the most adaptive man, who patterns his behavior on a successful analysis of the situation and unfailingly chooses the course of action best fitted to bring about the result he wishes, then clearly such an emotional bias would reduce the range of his adaptiveness, for he would be impelled at times by emotional responses such as fear or anger, to follow an ill-chosen course.

Currently there are serious questions as to whether man's

inventive capacity may not be transforming the world so rapidly as to be outrunning even his adaptive powers. Our study is concerned, however, not with the improvement of technology in dealing with the physical world, but with the improvement of techniques in dealing with the *human* world and, more fundamentally, with the improvement of human interactions and exchanges so that man, who has become dominant as a species, can be fulfilled as an individual.

The great advantage of learning, in the control of behavior, over the rigidly pre-set behavior we see in the instinctual behavior of insects, is that learned behavior is so much more flexible. It does not require countless generations of biological selection to change it, but it can be changed by behavioral invention and stabilized by education.

Every human society shapes its members for social living with one another. The learning of trust is followed by the learning of communication. Human society, even in its simplest forms, sets complex requirements upon the individual. This is certainly true of our own society, with which we are most familiar.

Let us consider an American university student who, at noon, finds himself hungry. Food is provided for his nourishment, but with the requirement of his conformity to a complicated set of requirements. He must seek out the cateteria, go to the end of the line, and in his turn collect tray, knife, fork, and spoon, paper napkin, proceed down the line, make his selections of food, pay the cashier, carry his selection on his tray to a table, and there eat according to a rigidly prescribed routine with knife, fork, and spoon. To neglect any of these prescribed details may damage his social standing, and to neglect payment may even bring him into conflict with the law.

The process of socialization is in great part learning to harmonize the inner needs and drives with the outer expectations of society. This harmony of behavior proceeds most easily when there is a reasonable harmony of emotional response behind it— that is, *when the individual genuinely cares about and is in empathy with his fellows.* This in turn appears to relate in large part to his early experiences.

It does appear that the early non-verbal communication of

the infant with his mother is of great importance to the development of his capacity for empathy and fellow-feeling with others. If his cries of distress bring not only the assuaging of his hunger or a soft clean dry diaper, but some gentle stimulation and rocking and gradually a rewarding interpersonal communication, he gradually develops his human capacity for feeling-with, for rapport.

Nothing is more important for the social adjustment of a human being than the development of a capacity to feel empathy with his fellows.

A Formulation of the Problem

In the ensuing pages we are to consider the behavior *disorders* of childhood and adolescence. A behavior disorder might be defined as *a persistent tendency toward some type of behavior inappropriate to the situation in which the individual finds himself.* Such inappropriate behavior tends to be repetitive and represents in a sense a restriction in the individual's range of appropriate behavior.

We can recognize two kinds of predispositions which tend either to limit the individual in the selection of an appropriate response or to push him toward the selection of an inappropriate response. One is biological and constitutional. The other is largely social and experiential.

The Biological Basis

Some physiologically-minded philosophers down the ages have mused at the relation of body form and personality. The ancient Chinese god of happiness, Ho Ti, is a fat figure with a body architecture like that of the jolly old St. Nick of our culture. It is reputed to bring good luck to rub the belly of Ho Ti. It is no accident that both Ho Ti and St. Nicholas are pictured with round bellies.

Twenty-four hundred years ago, Hippocrates, the father of medicine, recognized the significance of body form in disease and described the apoplectic type and the phthisical type. Kretschmer[31], in the present century, was impressed with the frequency of what he called the pyknic habitus in manic-depressive disease as compared with schizophrenia, and built a system on the correspondence of the pyknic habitus and extroversion as compared with introversion. George Draper[2], in the Constitution Clinic at Columbia University, contrasted the body form characteristic of peptic ulcer patients with that characteristic of patients with gall bladder disease. It remained for W. H. Sheldon[42] to supply a logical and, more specifically, an embryological basis for the relation of physique and character.

Sheldon rationalizes his body types in terms of the three embryonal layers—endoderm, mesoderm, and ectoderm—and "somatotypes" each individual in terms of the prominence of these layers in his developed body—the degree of his endomorphy, his mesomorphy, and his ectomorphy.

Endomorphs, of whom Ho Ti and St. Nicholas are conspicuous examples, are characterized by the predominance of the endoderm, which gives rise to the digestive system. These individuals tend to be big-bellied and fat. Sheldon describes their typical traits as viscerotonic. They are food-loving, pleasure-loving, sociable, and companionable. The last word betrays its origin. A companion is literally one with whom one breaks bread (*com panis*).

Bone and muscles develop from the mesoderm, and mesomorphs are square and muscular. Sheldon describes their typical traits as somatotonic—bold, adventurous, assertive, aggressive, endowed with a love of action.

The third layer is the ectoderm, from which the brain, the eyes and the skin develop. Sheldon describes the typical traits of the ectomorph as cerebrotonic. He is sensitive, thoughtful, inhibited, and shy. He seeks an intellectual rather than a social or aggressive solution to problems.

While the correlations between body form and these behavioral tendencies are not high, yet there are correlations. Certainly experience is likely to reinforce any such constitutional tendencies. Aggressive behavior is more likely to pay off if you have a good musculature than if you do not, and body form certainly does create some predispositions.

More recently, the longitudinal studies of Alexander Thomas and his co-workers[46] have made it clear that there are temperamental consistencies of behavior which develop very early in life and which seem not accountable in terms of parental handling or management. These temperamental characteristics, moreover, are significantly related to the development of clinical problems.[47] The level of predictive validation is presently low, but is definitely beyond chance.

The Experiential Basis

The remainder of this book is largely concerned with the characterological basis of generally observed patterns of maladjustment. Such a characterological basis can certainly not exclude biological elements such as mesomorphy, but it is much more concerned with differences of experience, especially *early* experience.

CHAPTER 2

A WORD ON METHOD

THE TRADITIONAL METHOD OF INVESTIGATION IN CHILD PSYCHIATRY, AS IN ADULT PSYCHIATRY, HAS BEEN THE INTENSIVE STUDY OF INDIVIDUAL CASES. THIS METHOD HAS BEEN EXTREMELY USEFUL IN CLINICAL WORK IN THE DEVELOPMENT OF A SENSE OF UNDERSTANDING ON WHICH TREATMENT EFFORTS CAN BE BASED. IT HAS BEEN PRODUCTIVE IN HYPOTHESES—BOTH HYPOTHESES ABOUT THE INDIVIDUAL CASE AND MORE GENERAL HYPOTHESES ABOUT THE USUAL DYNAMICS OF SUCH CASES. HOWEVER, IT HAS BEEN OF A VERY LIMITED VALUE IN THE VERIFICATION OF GENERAL HYPOTHESES. CONFIDENCE IN THE GENERALITY OF A RELATIONSHIP—FOR EXAMPLE, BETMEEN A BACKGROUND FACTOR AND A PERSONALITY ELEMENT— IS NOT GREATLY INCREASED BY FINDING THAT THE RELATIONSHIP WHICH EXISTS IN ONE CASE EXISTS IN TWO CASES, NOR EVEN THAT THE RELATIONSHIP FOUND IN BOTH OF THE TWO CASES MAY BE FOUND IN 100 PER CENT OF FOUR CASES.

For verification of general hypotheses, it is necessary to test the constancy of relations. Since we deal with almost no relations which are invariable, these tests are necessarily statistical. It has often been very difficult for child psychiatrists to accept or to admit to the limited and dubious state of our knowledge, but illusions and professional defensiveness do not lead to professional growth. The tools of scientific investigation must be cultivated in psychiatry if our field is to advance. Interpretive case study and statistical logic must be combined in order to insure our progress in this direction. Statistical method is not an alternative to case study. It is simply a scientific method for controlling or estimating the effect of random variance. Moreover, since the uncontrolled factors with which we deal are always large, it is necessary to our field.

Incidentally, clinical judgments and statistical methods are supplementary, not contrasting. Clinical judgments of experts in our field can be quantified and treated statistically.

Statistical method makes it possible to focus on one relationship at a time, either to verify or disprove a general hypothesis arrived at clinically, or to define relationships which call for clinical study and clinical explanation.

This book is born in part *from years of clinical work with children* and in part *from statistical analyses of bodies of data* on clinical cases. These are supplementary methods. *Both* are necessary for effective synthesis in the field of child psychiatry at present.

It may not be surprising to the reader that the product which arises from such synthesis is humanly quite understandable, in that it bears obvious and important relations to our ancient human knowledge of human beings and human society. Systems of seeking to understand human behavior which find it necessary to begin by replacing the learner's human understanding with de-humanizing technical jargon, at best take the learner on a time-consuming detour. Our human understanding certainly does need to be extended. It certainly should not be discarded.

The effort to promote the adjustment of maladjusted children has gone on from time immemorial, and when parents have been concerned about their children's behavior and have not been successful in normalizing or controlling it, they have sought professional help from religion, from education, from psychology, and from the field of medicine. Despite the fact that libraries of information, suggestions and advice have been written, still, what with the elusiveness and complexity of human behavior and human interaction, parents are seeking professional guidance with respect to problems which they are not able to master or even to manage.

Interpreting Group Statistics

In considering the amount of effort that has gone into this field, it is surprising that there has been so little study which has involved grouping and classification of behavior disorders and which has then sought to find *common background factors* among those disorders which appear to be behaviorally related. From this point of view, the present study is simply an effort to determine the characteristics of the distinguishable behavioral groups and then to seek the concomitant factors which are related to these.

It must be admitted that the statistical study of these behavior groups needs to be interpreted with a measure of caution, for otherwise this method does carry with it some dangers of promoting false conclusions. For example, we have found that the stability of the families of retarded children who are brought to the clinic appears to be above the clinic average. This does not justify a judgment that stable families are more likely to have retarded children than unstable families. That would be a quite unwarranted conclusion. The explanation lies rather with the selective factors which bring children to the clinic. Mental retardation is such a severe handicap that it brings children to the clinic regardless of other factors. That is to say, mentally retarded children have a severe handicap from birth and are brought to a clinic regardless of the family stability.

By contrast, children of normal intelligence are not likely to be brought to the clinic unless they show behavior problems. But such children are much more likely to develop behavior problems (and consequently to be brought to the clinic) if the family is unstable. The clinic is not so likely to have referred to it children of normal intelligence from stable families. Thus, the selective factor which brings mentally retarded children to the clinic *whether the family is stable or unstable* but which is likely to bring children of normal intelligence to the clinic *only if the family is unstable* artificially builds into the clinic population a positive correlation between mental retardation in the child and family stability. This correlation is an artifact of the manner of selection of the clinic population.

Stated another way, the effect of the selective process is such that if two elements, A and B, are *uncorrelated* in the general population and both are reasons for the referral to the clinic, then we may expect that A and B will be *negatively correlated* in the clinic population. This should make us very cautious about assuming that the instance of a negative correlation between items such as A and B in the clinic population is an indication that items A and B will be negatively correlated in the population at large or that the absence of A causes B.

Methods of Clustering and the Clusters

The present work began with an effort by Lester Hewitt[4] to verify the existence, in a clinic population of 500 cases from the Michigan Child Guidance Institute, of three types of delinquents I had described from clinical observations in a training school for delinquent boys and to verify the particular family backgrounds I had hypothesized for each. The following quotation is from my paper "Child Relationships and Delinquency and Crime" in Reckless, "The Etiology of Delinquent and Criminal Behavior."[37]

There is much evidence that the role of the family in early life, the interpersonal relationships, and the dynamics of the family group have an important determining part in personality formation. There is evidence to support the view that they have an important determining role with respect ot many instances of delinquency and crime, which are, like other human acts, an expression of the personality in its attempt at adaptation. The following hypotheses are suggested for research test:

1. The aggressive delinquent with hostile, bitter, hardened attitudes, little in the way of standards, a lack of guilt sense, and a pattern of viewing himself as the victim, even when he is the aggressor, is usually a child rejected from birth, and having never known a normal child-parent relationship. His own sense of deprivation is the focus of attention for this delinquent to a degree which effectively protects him from seeing his acts as they appear to others.

2. The loyal member of a delinquent gang, the good comrade of a delinquent sub-culture, has usually experienced a more or less adequate child-parent relationship in early childhood but through a deficiency of interests, supervision, or control on the part of his parents in late childhood and adolescence, has essentially lost

effective emotional rapport with the adult world and lives almost exclusively, from a social point of view, with his small delinquent group. The gang member typically comes from a family of several children.

3. The "con-man" type of personality who deliberately works himself into the confidence of others for the purpose of exploiting that confidence to his own gain frequently develops in a situation of parental disharmony where he is essentially a pawn in the conflict, and is under the necessity of developing, for his own protection, the ability to play off one parent against the other. Neither parent has been dependable enough to give him real trust, and his early experiences have required that he develop skill in manipulating others.

Entries from the fairly extensive case records available on the 500 cases were coded and punched on IBM cards and a search was made for the three clusters, without benefit of a computer, as such help was not then available. There was no problem in finding a cluster of unsocialized aggressive children and a cluster of gang delinquents. The "con man" type of personality was too infrequent to constitute a cluster in our limited material. A third group which was obvious were the inhibited children. The results of this study were published.[4, 27] These initial groupings of traits for the selection of groups were done not by statistical method, but "free hand" by clinical judgment somewhat guided by the degree of association between selected traits.

A further step was to examine the clusters of correlated traits which could be found in the extensive material of 5,000 clinic cases published from the Institute for Juvenile Research by Luton Ackerson.[1] Correlations were tested separately for over 2,000 boys and over 1,000 girls.

Our procedure was to begin with each of the hundred-odd traits listed and add the trait with which it correlated most highly. Then the third trait added was the one which had the highest correlation with the first two, the fourth trait added was the one which had the highest correlation with the first three, and so on. In this way the approach to the clustering was wholly objective and was in no way dependent on the preconceptions of the investigator.

This procedure applied to the intercorrelation of the traits of the 2,113 boys led to three major clusters.[25] These major clusters were identified as the socialized delinquent, the unsocialized aggressive boy and the overinhibited boy. When we proceeded in the same fashion with the intercorrelation of the traits of 1,118 girls, three closely corresponding clusters were obtained.

By slightly altering the requirements, it was possible to increase the number of clusters from three to five for both the boys and girls. This alteration was simply to add the rule that if a trait were common to two clusters, it would not be used for the selection of additional traits for either cluster. This simple change made it possible with both the boys and the girls to include a cluster relating to the brain-injured child and a cluster relating to the schizoid child. It also resulted in a second slightly variant group of unsocialized aggressive girls, who showed a high level of verbal aggression.

A more recent study in Japan by Kobayashi, Mizushima and Shinohara[30] demonstrated four major clusters among 200 boys 6 to 16 years of age judged to be problem children in child guidance centers in Tokyo. The best-marked symptom cluster they identified with the socialized delinquent child; the second best marked cluster was the unsocialized aggressive child; and the third was the overinhibited child. They listed a fourth "unstable" type, which corresponds with the hyperkinetic reaction.

Obviously, the nature of clusters found will depend upon the nature of the traits included. If traits representative of one of these clusters are not included, the cluster will not be found. A clinic population is by definition a selected population, and the size of correlations will be influenced by specific factors relating to *how* the selection is made.

The foregoing methods produced *clusters of correlated traits.* An alternative method involves the clustering of *individuals* on the basis of their resemblance one to another. This has been done by computer. The symptoms of each case were punched on an IBM card and each card was grouped with the card it resembled most. This created clusters, but the fact that each card was placed with *the card it resembled most* did not insure that it was in the *group* it resembled most. Proceeding from the initial groups, the average resemblance of each card to all the other cards in its cluster was calculated, as was its average resemblance to each card in each of the other clusters. Those cards having a greater average resemblance to the cards in another cluster than to the cards in the cluster to which they were initially assigned, were re-assigned, and the process was repeated until the groups stabilized.

This method was applied to the 500 cases from the Michigan Child Guidance Institute.[12] The program accommodated only 125 cards at a time. Some initial groups disappeared as a result of the process of re-assigning cards. This left us with four parallel sets of groups, each set from clustering 125 cards. One card was then punched to represent the characteristics of each group and by a repetition of the clustering procedure, this time clustering groups, we came out with five master groups. It was clear that our original three groups were all here—the socialized delinquent, the unsocialized aggressive and an overinhibited or overanxious group. We found ourselves also with a shy-seclusive group which resembled the schizoid group found in Ackerson's material, and with a hyperkinetic group which resembled behaviorally the brain-damaged group from Ackerson's material.

A more recent clustering[14, 15] of the 1,500 cases from the IJR (Institute for Juvenile Research) came up with the same five groups—the socialized delinquents, the unsocialized aggressive, the overanxious, the withdrawing and, an organic-hyperkinetic group. These are essentially the same major clusters.

Interpreting Correlations

Such statistical measures depend upon the use of a checklist or rating scale. The problems of using a rating scale or checklist include one's tendency toward multiplying the scales in order to get a more complete description of the patient. This can be carried to the point which makes the study bog down because of the excessively large number of scales. Efforts may be made to avoid this by groupings of composite scales. This was done in the collection of data at the Institute for Juvenile Research. Most of these combination scales were quite satisfactory, as it is a description of the mother's attitude toward the child as *critical, depreciative* or a description of a child's relationship with the psychologist as *shy, withdrawn, inhibited.* A special feature sometimes recorded in the psychiatric interview, *motor restlessness* or *incoordination,* is less satisfactory, for while restlessness and incoordination may exist together with a common cause, they may also exist independently and for different reasons. Their relationship becomes blurred in such a composite scale.

Occasionally one may have a real problem in interpreting a positive correlation with a composite scale in which different items with different meanings have been included. In the grouping together of *maternal character disturbance* and *maternal psychoneurosis,* for example, one wonders if the ensuing unsocialized aggressive reaction is occasioned by its being related to maternal character disturbance and *not* by any relation between it and maternal psychoneurosis. However, the correlation itself can give no clue as to which item is related.

When one has demonstrated the existence of a cluster and wishes to compare statistically a group of cases which fit the cluster with cases which do not, a useful method is to select cases which show more than one of the traits in the cluster. The more traits required, the more purely the selected group of cases exemplify the cluster; but, of course, the smaller the group, the larger the effect of random variance. For as a group becomes smaller, chance factors play a larger role. If a group of traits is highly correlated and widely distributed, more selective requirements can be introduced without reducing the size of the group too much. In the studies on which this book is largely founded, I have required two to four traits for inclusion of a case, depending on the circumstances.

This study is in part based on material hitherto unpublished, particularly in relation to the 1,500 Institute for Juvenile Research cases referred to earlier.

CHAPTER 3

THE MENTALLY ILL AND THE CLASSIFICATION OF PSYCHIATRIC DISORDERS

EVERY SOCIETY HAS HAD THE PROBLEM OF DEALING WITH THOSE WHOSE MINDS ARE GROSSLY DISORDERED. THE METHOD CHOSEN BEARS A RELATION TO THE CONCEPTUAL EXPLANATION OF MENTAL DISORDER, WHICH IS DOMINANT IN THAT SOCIETY. WHEN MENTAL DISORDER WAS VIEWED AS DEMON POSSESSION, EFFORTS WERE DIRECTED TOWARD EXORCIZING OR BANISHING THE EVIL SPIRITS FROM THE PERSON WHO WAS VIEWED AS "POSSESSED." OFTEN IN THESE ZEALOUS EFFORTS TO DRIVE OUT THE EVIL SPIRIT, DISCRIMINATION BECAME CLOUDED, AND CRUEL METHODS WERE EMPLOYED UPON THE PATIENT HIMSELF.

A humanitarian culture is put under great strain by individuals who, because of mental disorder, cannot be prevailed to act in ways deemed appropriate. A common solution has been banishment. Primitive societies might banish the individual into the forest, but as the forests receded, this became more and more difficult. The ancient Greeks banished the mentally ill to waterless islands in the Aegean, supplying them periodically with food and drink.

Early in the nineteenth century, mental hospitals in America depended on the application of what was called the moral treatment, which in effect, through structured activities and kindly direction at the human, interpersonal level, simply sought to develop the best potentialities of the patient. This method of treatment had a very substantial level of success.

The expansion of the mental hospital resulted in the impersonality of mass care. The per diem cost of state hospital care remained the same while wages rose sharply, and the cost of the care in the general hospital rose even more sharply. The discoveries in bacteriology focused attention on the microscope, but the "schizococcus" or bacterium presumed to cause schizophrenia has never been found. During the latter part of the nineteenth century and the earliest years of the twentieth, the mental hospital gradually deteriorated from a place of humane treatment and of hope to a place of banishment, which served the limited purpose of protecting society from the embarrassment occasioned by the presence of the mentally ill in its midst.

While the mental hospital was retrogressing in this way to the rather inhumane solution of mere custodial detention, the creative mind of Sigmund Freud was making some discoveries and gradually finding an understanding of psychodynamics—chiefly through the study of psychoneurotic individuals, usually the victims of anxiety and inner conflict. These patients often recognized the illogicality of some of their ideas and impulses and did not permit their grip on objective reality to crumble. The work of Freud was accepted by only a few of his medical contemporaries, but his methods of treatment enjoyed a degree of success and attracted non-medical professional followers, as well as a great deal of popular interest. As a result, psychoanalysis opened doors for many and yet continued to develop in isolation, acquiring many of the characteristics of a closed system of faith. This made its incorporation into the general field of psychiatry difficult. The new discoveries, however, served to focus attention on those mental disorders short of psychosis, and to promote an interest in the field of non-psychotic mental illness. Thus the work of Freud has had a profound effect on psychiatry and has done more to create a respect for and understanding of psychodynamics than any other historical development.

Diagnosis means literally *a knowledge through and through.* Diagnosis, as it is commonly used, includes the asisgnment of the patient's illness to a specific category. Such assignment, hopefully, will reflect the treatment indicated and the prognosis.

It has often been emphasized that "every case is individual," and this is undeniably true. It is also true that we can learn from one case to another only as we recognize similarities and differences, and this soon involves categorizing the cases in some way. Such categorizing is a simple form of classification or diagnosis, and thus any differential understanding in this area depends upon some type of diagnostic classification.

If we take an example from another field of medicine, *meningitis* refers to an inflammation of the meninges. The further identification and inclusion of the offending organism in the diagnoses *tuberculous meningitis* or *meningococcus meningitis* determine specific antibiotic treatment and affect the prognosis enormously. At its best, diagnosis definitively determines treatment. This happy situation obtains when we have adequate treatment methods for the particular condition diagnosed, as is often the case when antibiotics are involved.

There are other situation in which diagnosis may disclose prognosis but have very little to offer by way of treatment, as in Tay-Sachs disease, or *amaurotic family idiocy*. Even here, where we have at present no effective treatment, diagnosis may determine prognosis and may make effective prevention possible.

The field of psychiatry includes mental disorders which are a result of organic illness, as in the delirium states or "support disorders." It includes mental disorders occasioned by organic disease of the brain, as in paresis. It also includes many mental disorders which occur with the brain organically intact, so far as our present methods of investigations are able to determine. It includes psychoses such as schizophrenia, which have, at least superficially, in the chronic state, many of the earmarks of an organic disorder, even though no organic pathology has yet been demonstrated. It includes the psychoneuroses, which may be demonstrably related to psychodynamics and which have sometimes demonstrated psychological contagion, as in the dancing mania of the Middle Ages and in the occasional outbreak of hysteria which has been recorded in girls' schools.

Thus the definition of mental illness has traditionally included both organic and functional disorders. The inclusion of the latter has been challenged by Thomas Szasz[44] who has proclaimed "mental illness" a myth.

It must be admitted that for the most part our knowledge of etiology and of treatment in psychiatric disorders is far from definitive. However, in medicine we have rarely seen treatment or prevention run ahead of diagnosis. While the clarification of a diagnostic problem certainly does not insure the development of effective treatment measures, it certainly makes their development much more likely.

Types of Classification

The clearest and most ancient distinction in the field of psychiatry is between those individuals whose mental state is grossly disordered and those whose mental state is either within or near the normal range. This distinction is humanly and administratively very important, for it marks the difference between the patient who is able to care for himself and the patient who, by reason of his disability, must be cared for by others. Psychoses were among the first recognized mental disorders and, because of the public problem they presented, were banished to the madhouse. It is doubtless for this historical reason that in the International Classification of Diseases, the primary distinction is between psychoses and non-psychotic mental disorders.

The 1952 Diagnostic and Statistical Manual of Mental Disorders of the American Psychiatric Association (DSM-I) represented a sharp departure from this history. Under the leadership of Dr. George Raines, the Association's Committee on Nomenclature and Statistics undertook to develop a nosology based upon etiological factors. In this they were influenced by the experience of the armed forces in World War II, and by the systems of nomenclature which had been proposed in the armed forces during that conflict. The primary division in this system of classification is between those diagnoses which are caused by or associated with impairment of brain tissue function and those which are not. That is to say, the primary distinction is between those disorders which are known or presumed to be organic, and those which are known or assumed to be functional.

In a number of ways, this classification represented an advance. For example, the fundamental etiological unity of the mental disorders associated with cerebral arteriosclerosis was recognized, whether or not the patient was simply forgetful or was disoriented and psychotic. However, in the area of functional disorders, the disorder is somehow an interaction between the individual and his environment. Under such circumstances, it is difficult to assign the etiology of the disorder to *either* the individual *or* to his envronment. The course usually followed was to ascribe essentially to environmental causes, disorder precipitated by environmental changes. These were put down as "transient situational disturbances," defined as follows:

> This general classification should be restricted to reactions which are more or less transient in character and which appear to be an acute symptom response to a situation, without apparent underlying personality disturbance.
>
> The symptoms are the immediate means used by the individual in his struggle to adjust to an overwhelming situation. In the presence of good adaptive capacity, recession of symptoms generally occurs when the situational stress diminishes. Persistent failure to resolve will indicate a more severe underlying disturbance and will be classified elsewhere.

What this discussion does not state is that, with the persistence of external pressure and resultant maladaptive response, the pattern of the maladaptive response gradually becomes more and more ingrained, more and more internalized. Most of the problems we see in children *begin* as situational reactions. That is to say, in most psychiatric problems we see in children, if one traces back the history, one will come to a point at which the diagnosis of an *adjustment reaction* would have been justified.

An extremely common adjustment reaction of childhood may be occasioned in the toddler by the arrival of a new baby in the family. If the toddler has recently achieved toilet training, there is very often a relapse. Probably in most instances such a relapse results from an increase in the toddler's level of anxiety, with a consequent reduction in bladder control. Occasionally it may be on the conscious level and relate to a direct jealousy of the attention given in diapering the new baby. If, however, the parental response to the toddler's enuresis is one of strong disapproval or punishment, the insecurity of the toddler may be increased, and a more morbid element of internalization of the problem may be promoted.

One of the disadvantages of DSM-I was that its categories were recognized by no organization except the American Psychiatric Association. The National Institute of Mental Health had to translate the diagnostic categories into those of the International Classification of Diseases before reporting them to the World Health Organization. Even the American Medical Association utilized the categories of this International Classification rather than those of the American Psychiatric Association.

For the preparation of the Revised Diagnostic and Statistical Manual of the A.P.A. (DSM-II), there was an organized effort to bridge this gap and build an acceptable compromise.

I.

One of the problems of classification has related to the lack of consistency in the use of the word "psychosis." Originally it refered to a sweeping disorder which approximated the lay term "crazy" or the legal term "insane." It was given to those disorders which often created such a degree of disturbance. Since, however, most mental disease is recoverable, and the milder and convalescent degrees of disorder were included, many persons with "psychoses" were not greatly disordered.

DSM-II has endeavored to resolve this problem by reserving the adjective *psychotic* for those individuals who are, at the time, grossly disordered.

> Patients are described as psychotic when their mental functioning is sufficiently impaired to interfere grossly with their capacity to meet the ordinary demands of life. The impairment may result from a serious distortion in their capacity to recognize reality. Hallucinations and delusions, for example, may distort their perceptions. Alternations of mood may be so profound that the patient's capacity to respond appropriately is grossly impaired. Deficits in perception, language, and memory may be so severe that the patient's capacity for mental grasp of his situation is effectively lost.
>
> Some confusion results from the different meanings which have

become attached to the word psychosis. Some non-organic disorders 295-298), in the well-developed form in which they were first recognized, typically rendered patients psychotic. For historical reasons, these disorders are still classified as psychoses, even though it now generally is recognized that many patients for whom these diagnoses are clinically justified are not in fact psychotic. This is true particularly in the incipient or convalescent stages of the illness. To reduce confusion, when one of these disorders listed as a "psychosis" is diagnosed in a patient who is not psychotic, the qualifying phrase *not psychotic* or *not presently psychotic* should be noted and coded .x6 with a fifth digit.

Example: 295.06 *Schizophrenia, simple type, not psychotic.*

It should be noted that this Manual permits an organic condition to be classified as a psychosis only if the patient is psychotic during the episode being diagnosed.

Since DSM-I had called to attention the continuity of disorder with cerebral arteriosclerosis from slight memory loss to frank psychosis, and since most of the international representatives working on a revision of the International Classification of Diseases were not willing to give up as a first division the administratively important dstinction between psychoses and non-psychotic conditions, the method used was to introduce into the Eighth Revision of the ICD a series of mental disorders associated with physical conditions but not specified as *psychotic*. Thus, if an old man should come into the hospital, not psychotic but with memory failure and some symptoms of second childhood as a result of arteriosclerosis, the diagnosis would be *non-psychotic organic brain syndrome with circulatory disturbance.* If, in the middle of the night, he became disoriented, hallucinated, and delusional, from the same cause, the diagnosis would be changed to *psychosis with cerebral arteriosclerosis.* This would remain the diagnosis for the remainder of this episode of illness, regardless of the disappearance of the psychotic symptoms.

II.

In addition to the psychoses, there is a second large group of disorders of more limited or topical nature, the psychoneuroses, which are known or presumed to result from anxiety or inner conflict. (We assign the word *fear* to a state of apprehension which is a response to a perceived outer threat to the integrity of the body. When the apprehension is in response to a more vague threat or a threat to the integrity of the mind, we call it *anxiety.*)

Inner conflicts occasion anxiety. Inner conflicts may be temporarily resolved by neurotic illness. For example, conversion hysteria represents the conversion of inner conflict into physical symptoms such as paralysis, blindness, or deafness. The common psychoneuroses are the direct expression of anxiety, either as anxiety or depression, or its conversion into physical symptoms or disabilities, or excessive preoccupation with defenses against anxiety, as in the obsessive-compulsive neurosis.

The psychoses forced themselves upon public attention very early. The common explanation was demon possession. The recognition of the psychoneuroses came later, but in the case of hysteria at least, the explanation of demon possession was also accepted initially. In a celebrated case in 1685, Soeur Jeanne des Anges, a Mother Superior of 28 years in Loudon, France, whose request to a handsome young priest that he become spiritual advisor to her nunnery had been rejected, accused him of contracting with the devil to bring about the diabolic possession of her and her nuns. On the basis of the record, the picture of hysteria seems quite clear, but the unfortunate Father Grandier was burned alive as a result of this accusation.

The confusion between the psychoneuroses and the organic disorders which they often mimic, is often quite difficult to unravel.

Psychophysiological disorders involve a large psychological contribution to what are, as a result, often in part organic disorders. In these cases the pathogenic effects appear to be mediated through the autonomic nervous system and the primitive smooth muscle of the organs, not subject to voluntary control.

III.

In addition to the psychoses and the psychoneuroses, there are recognized in psychiatry the personality disorders. "This group of disorders is characterized by deeply ingrained maladaptive patterns of behavior that are perceptibly different in quality from psychotic and neurotic symptoms. Generally these are life-long patterns, often recognizable by the time of adolescence or earlier."

That is to say, a diagnosis of a personality disorder simply tells us that the individual so diagnosed has a characteristic repetitive (and maladaptive) pattern of reactions in daily life. When, for whatever reason, what may have begun as a transient situational reaction becomes internalized and crystallized in a deeply ingrained repetitive maladaptive pattern, then we are dealing with a personality disorder. DSM-II describes ten common personality disorders and allows a miscellaneous category of other specified types of personality disorders. Three of these disorders resemble major psychoses, although the patient is not psychotic. These are *paranoid personality, cyclothymic personality,* and *schizoid personality.* A fourth disorder* *inadequate personality* resembles mental deficiency even though the patient is not mentally deficient.

Four of the personality disorders listed in DSM-II resemble psychoneuroses.** These are *obsessive-compulsive personality, hysterical personality, asthenic personality,* and *passive-aggressive personality.*

The *passive-aggressive personality,* like the *inadequate personality,* is retained in DSM-II from DSM-I even though neither was included in ICD-8. Whenever—as in any occupied country— individuals are confronted by authority they resent and wish to resist, but do not dare challenge openly, we see passive-aggressive behavior. Orders are misunderstood or somehow carried out in a way that defeats their purpose. Work progress is slow, and matters somehow get disorganized. Such passive-aggressive behavior is purposeful and may be "functional" in achieving its purpose under such circumstances. If so, we cannot reasonably classify it as maladaptive. When, however, passive-aggressive

---

* These four resembling psychoses or mental deficiency were grouped in DSM-I under the heading *personality pattern disturbances.*

** In DSM-I there was no *asthenic personality.* *Obsessive-compulsive personality* has replaced the *compulsive personality* of DSM-I and the *emotionally unstable personality* of that volume is replaced by *hysterical* personality. These changes are in accord with ICD-8.

behavior becomes a characteristic way of behaving *regardless of whether or not it is contributing to a reasonable goal,* we may reasonably classify it as maladaptive. Where the psychoneurotic has an inner conflict, the passive-aggressive has a conflict between an outer requirement and an inner resistance. When this mode of reaction is not a selective response to specific external situations but has become a characteristic and generalized response of the individual, he may be classified as a *passive-aggressive personality.*

The *antisocial personality* describes a basically unsocialized personality who lives in society. He lacks loyalty, and since morality begins with loyalty, he lacks morality.

The *explosive personality* is a new entry in DSM-II: it is applicable to a person strongly predisposed to outbursts of rage strikingly different from his usual behavior.

After the personality disorders, DSM-II lists the sexual deviations, then alcoholism, and drug dependence, the psychophysiological disorders already referred to, and special symptoms. The last elements of DSM-II, the transient situational disturbances, the behavior disorders of childhood and adolescence, and the conditions without manifest psychiatric disorder will be discussed in Chapter 5.

CHAPTER 4

THE INITIAL STUDY

AN EARLIER PUBLICATION IN COLLABORATION WITH LESTER HEWITT[27] STATED SO WELL THE APPROACH ON INITIAL FINDINGS OF OUR FIRST VENTURE INTO TYPE-TRACKING THAT IT IS HERE QUOTED AT LENGTH WITH SLIGHT REVISION OF TERMINOLOGY TO FIT THE CURRENT OFFICIAL DIAGNOSTIC MANUAL.

Scientific progress in child psychiatry depends, as in other fields, upon reducing the infinite variety of problems through some broad conceptualization. It goes without saying that any schematization involves some oversimplification and hence some distortion. The justification for any scheme depends upon the aid it gives to understanding the phenomena represented. In presenting our scheme of personality structure, we believe we are emphasizing concepts which are useful and valuable in child psychiatry. We are fully aware that our scheme is not exhaustive, that all cases cannot be fitted into the scheme and that a tremendous amount of significant material about the individual case is ignored. Our description of these types is a compounding of tendencies that are typical. No case may fit the scheme perfectly. The case is a particular reality and the scheme is an abstraction. One should never make the mistake of treating the scheme as a reality. Rather, the scheme should aid in understanding the reality of the individual case. If this scheme contributes to the understanding of many maladjusted children, it will have accomplished its purpose.

While major elements in the scheme are frankly taken over from Freud, the concepts here presented are in themselves in no sense sectarian and will, it is hoped, be intelligible to all

28

who work in this field regardless of the question of sectarian identification.

The personality is conceived as having a central core of primitive impulses. Primitive is here used in the sense of spontaneous and socially undisciplined, or instinctual in the Freudian terminology. Around this core of primitive impulse there is in the adult or in the older child a shell of inhibition which prevents free expression of the impulses. This corresponds somewhat with the Freudian concept of superego, while the core of primitive impulses represents the Freudian concept of the id. This shell represents repressing forces which keep the primitive impulses unconscious and prevent them from coming into action, except as modified through social discipline.

The surface zone of the personality is the ego—conscious, socialized, discriminating, and choosing. It is our thesis that the three major types of personality structure encountered in child psychiatry may be illustrated by the three diagrams in Figure 1.

In Type I we see an individual who has an excessive development of the shell of inhibition. As a result of this the primitive impulses are denied adequate expression. Tension mounts within the personality and strong pressures develop in the struggle between the primitive impulses and the repressive forces. This individual is chronically in a state of internal conflict. Here we have the over-inhibited individual likely to react to these internal conflicts by developing terror dreams or anxiety attacks, or by developing physical symptoms of illness through conversion hysteria, or to defend himself from them by compulsive rituals. We do not, as a rule, see such well-developed neurotic symptoms in the child, but we see the milder over-inhibited symptoms of shyness, seclusiveness, fears, clinging, tics, sleep disturbances, nail biting, and other common evidences of tension and anxiety with which the child guidance worker is familiar. The essential points are to recognize that the person with severe internal conflict is, as a rule, the over-inhibited individual.

Type II represents the opposite of Type I. Type II represents the individual with an inadequate shell of internal inhibitions.

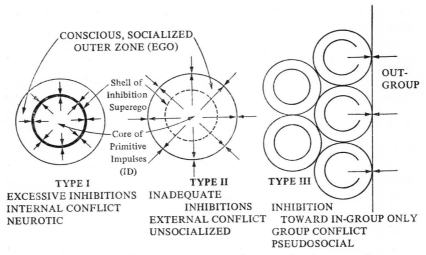

Figure 1.   Three Major Types of Personality Structure.*

As a result the primitive impulses come not only into consciousness but into expression very directly, providing there are no external pressures which check them. Such an individual is unsocialized and aggressive in his actions and is continually coming in conflict with others—the authorities and the police—as a result of his freely giving vent to his primitive impulses. This represents a type of personality totally different from Type I, although many workers who use terms loosely will speak of this unsocialized, aggressive type of individual as neurotic. It is our belief that such a usage leads to a confusion of thinking and of treatment and that the expression should not be used for this type of personality which allies itself rather with the psychopathic personality of asocial and amoral character.

Type III represents a more nearly normal type of personality structure than either of the foregoing. There is a normal shell of inhibition toward members of an in-group. Toward members of any out-group there is a deficit in the inhibitions, no sense of

---

* This diagram originally appeared in an article by R. L. Jenkins and L. Hewitt, entitled "Types of Personality Structure Encountered in Child Guidance Clinics" (*American Journal of Orthopsychiatry*, Vol. 14, 1944). Copyright, The American Orthopsychiatric Association, Inc. Reproduced by permission.

obligation and a free expression of the primitive impulses. In child guidance we see here the boy showing the group delinquent reaction, the loyal gang member, the good comrade of the delinquent subculture who is socialized—often highly socialized—within a delinquent group but regards the rest of the world as fair prey.

Our study of these types of personality structure is supported by an extensive and detailed statistical analysis of 500 cases examined at the Michigan Child Guidance Institute. The data cannot be presented here, and it will be necessary simply to indicate the general outline with a few bold strokes.

The overinhibited personality structure is extremely familiar to mental hygienists. Typically, it develops in an atmosphere of parental repression. The parents are likely to be cold and unsocial, the mother compensating for some rejection by overprotection and overrestriction, the father perfectionistic and intolerant. Both parents are inconsistent in methods of discipline. Both parents are restrained, socially disciplined persons. They are typically of a social stratum and a level of education above the clinic average. The mother is likely frequently to be ill from one affliction or another. The child himself is likely to have experienced an unusual amount of illness which contributes to his insecurity and dependence. He is likely to be jealous of his siblings in their relation to the parents, feeling his own relation less secure.

In order to understand such a personality structure, we need only to consider the dynamics of personality development. The young child obtains his sense of security from his parents; he has no other source of security. He is utterly dependent upon the parents, and there is no frequent childhood fear which produces such chronic anxiety as the fear of loss of the parents, or the fear of loss of parent love. Just as the parent is the fundamental source of security to the young child, fear of loss of the parents is the fundamental source of insecurity and of anxiety. This fact is so simple and obvious it is often overlooked.

Here we are dealing with the unsociable, cold, distant parent lacking in warmth. The child lacks the assurance, through close emotional contact with the parents, of acceptance and affection. These are parents whose approval (and presumably whose love) can be won only by very good, very conforming, very inhibited behavior. Any violation of parental taboos is met by disapproval which this insecure child feels or fears means rejection. There is deeply implanted, as the result of this experience, the pervading fear that if he is not a good child his parents will not love him. As a result, any aggressive act by the child throws him into a panic of anxiety. He can feel secure only by being excessively good, by being excessively inhibited. To protect himself he screws down the safety valve on his central core of primitive impulses, and the pressure there mounts to produce an acute situation of internal conflict, which may be relieved by neurotic disorders.

The Type II personality pattern is really simpler than Type I and might well have been presented first but for the fact that psychiatric and mental hygiene circles are more familiar with the overinhibited personality than with the unsocialized, aggressive type represented in Type II.

This child's problem centers around his uninhibited hostile treatment of others. He is cruel, defiant, prone deliberately to destroy the property of others as well as violently to attack their persons. He shows little feeling of guilt or remorse. He is seldom able to get along with other children, but is always quarreling, fighting or engaging in mischievous annoying tricks. He is inclined to bully and boss, and is boastful, selfish and jealous. He is rude or defiant toward persons in authority, openly antagonistic toward his teachers and has outbursts of temper when crossed. He will deceive others and refuses to accept the blame for his own misbehavior. Because of his personality makeup, he has few close friends, if any.

Even if others attempt to become friendly, this boy does not respond with friendship, for he is suspicious and reacts negatively. He is noncommittal and evasive when questioned and usually appears sullen. He seeks vengeance against those he dislikes. In our small series we find even arson and murder. Frequent petty thieving at home or at school sometimes results from the same vengeful attitude. His language is profane and obscene. He displays an unusually overt interest in sex, and *is known* to indulge in masturbation.

Typically, this boy lives in a deteriorated neighborhood, either in the country or at the edge of town. His troubles, however, did not begin in this neighborhood or even in this particular home, for his life has been very unstable. He has carried his troubles with him since birth and their origins even preceded this unhappy event, in the pre-marital experience of his parents. His mother's own home life in particular has been unhappy. It is likely that she left home at an early age to get away from her own parents and met the child's father. The child is likely to have been illegitimate.

In any event neither parent wanted the pregnancy and the mother was probably under considerable emotional strain during that period. Labor may have been prolonged or exceedingly difficult and, if so, the suffering the mother experienced only served to increase any existing tendency to reject the child. Both parents, but particularly the mother, denied this child affection from the beginning. Even if the parents married, desertion or divorce is likely to have broken the relationship, with the child being subsequently placed either temporarily or permanently with relatives or strangers or being shuttled from one parent to the other. If the parents remained together, their relationship was fraught with bitterness and disharmony. The mother is likely to have been very unstable, a characteristic not entirely foreign to her husband, who was also deceptive in his dealings with others. Both parents were probably violent-tempered and abusive toward each other or the children. The mother, possibly of low intelligence, may also have been addicted to the use of alcohol. She may have been and perhaps still is quite unwilling to accept the responsibilities of motherhood, and has frequently been involved in illicit sex affairs with various men. The family itself is regarded with disfavor by the neighbors and may be known unfavorably throughout the community.

No other relationships between the members of the family are encouraging to the development of a healthy social attitude on the part of the child. Rarely is authority in this family reasonably divided between the parents. One of them is usually extremely dominating and the other assumes little direct responsibility. The parents quarrel or engage in open fights and what loyalty exists between members of the family is split between opposing factional units. Sexual relationships between the parents are unsatisfactory and contribute to conflict. The status of the child in the home is also a source of conflict. The parents disagree on methods of discipline in which the father particularly is likely to be inconsistent.

The mother, and to a greater extent the father, will brook no interference from the outside, frequently shielding the child from the charges of school and community authorities. Neither parent, however, is affectionate toward him. They are at most indifferent in their attitudes and the mother is most likely to be openly hostile or rejecting. Little wonder then that he feels unwanted in the home and is ambivalent toward his parents or openly expresses hostility to parents and siblings alike.

In view of the mother's behavior, it is not surprising that other children in the home may also have engaged in unconventional sex behavior, and it is probable that one or more is officially known to the juvenile court as a delinquent on other counts. As a final note of emphasis, the picture presented is essentially one of generalized and continual parental rejection, and particularly overt maternal rejection, beginning at or before the birth of the child.

The product of this background is a child of bottomless hostilities and endless bitterness, who feels cheated in life, views himself as the victim although he is constantly the aggressor, is grossly defective in his social inhibitions, or if you prefer, in his superego, and is grossly lacking in guilt sense over his misconduct. We may think of his hostility as springing from three sources. First, there is the hostility of the individual who has a need for and, by common judgment, a right to expect love from his parents and receives none. Even adults who have developed a good deal of social restraint often become hostile and sometimes even violent when they find themselves rejected in a love relationship, and certainly the reaction of resentment and bitterness is natural to a child who is rejected by his mother. Secondly, this child has lacked an effective affectional tie to any adult through which he could incorporate standards of behavior or from whom he could develop a superego. In the third place, the example of behavior this child sees before him is one which is highly selfish and inconsiderate and, by our conventional standards, objectionable if not delinquent. This background has developed a hostile, uninhibited personality, tending to act with direct violence at any provocation or desire. He has cause for insecurity and cause for anxiety, but the anxiety usually leads him to attack.

Our third type of personality structure is not quite on a level with the other two, for it is the result of tendencies which developed at a higher level of differentiation. This is the group delinquent—the loyal gang member, the good comrade of a delinquent subculture. Within his own group he is commonly a socialized and adjusted individual. It is only in relation to the larger group that he can be considered maladjusted and antisocial.

While his behavior bears certain resemblances to that of the unsocialized, aggressive boy, there are important differences. These are related to the fact that he is socialized in his own group and loyal to his comrades. This boy also is deceptive and defiant toward authority. When possible he avoids self-incrimination by not accepting the blame for his own acts and he feels little guilt over his delinquent depredations. On the other hand, should he violate the code of his group, as by informing on his companions when caught, he would feel deeply guilty. Even more than the unsocialized, aggressive boy, he engages in petty stealing at home or school, but this behavior would appear to be motivated more by acquistiveness than by a desire for revenge. He also is extremely antagonistic toward school attendance, but expresses this antagonism chiefly in truancy. This antagonism to school is not due to lack of friends there, for compared with the average child seen at the clinic, this boy is popular.

He is engaged in a good deal of furtive stealing, either alone or in the company of others and is likely to have engaged in aggressive stealing as well. He is quite likely to be a member of some rather well-organized adolescent gang, and invariably is known to be associating with companions whom others consider to be undesirable and delinquent. He remains on the street late at night or may neglect to come home at all. He may be an inveterate smoker and probably has some experience in sex relations with girls. Among his own group he is "hail-fellow-well-met," but to the good people of the dominant society from whom he dissociates himself, he is a menace to law and order.

His home is located in a deteriorated downtown neighborhood where traditions of delinquency and disrespect for law are most likely to flourish. His family is held in disrepute even among such neighbors and offers little in the way of constructive training in conformity to rules of the larger society. His home is physically inadequate in every respect. The family is obliged to accept outside financial aid, or at least to confine its spending to bare necessities. The house is sadly in need of repair; it is crowded among other buildings so that little space is available for safe and supervised play at home. The interior of the home may be inadequately equipped with sanitary and other household facilities, and is in all probability unkempt. The family is a large one and four or more persons may be obliged to sleep in the same room—possibly three or more occupying the same bed. The boy is aware of and sensitive to the unfavorable contrast which his circumstances present in comparison with those of other children he knows.

Contrasted with the uninhibited aggressive boy, who represents a failure particularly of maternal function, expressed in overt maternal rejection, the group-delinquent boy represents typically a failure in paternal function—the neglect of supervision, training and control for the older child. The father's own childhood is much more likely to have been markedly unpleasant than is the mother's, and it is the father more than the mother in this case who has expressed subsequent unwillingness to accept family responsibilities. Both parents are inclined to be alcoholic, violent-tempered or abusive. The father may also have a reputation for dishonesty. The chronic illness or physical impairment which he may suffer reduces his effectiveness both as a breadwinner and as a parent. The siblings are likely to be known either officially or unofficially to the court as delinquents.

Between the members of the family there is likely to be disharmony which on the surface appears similar to that within the family of the rejected child. Both the expressions and implications of this disharmony, however, differ in a number of respects. There may be mutual indifference between the members of the family and little feeling of common interest or loyalty—there may be split loyalties with the possibility that the delinquent boy allies himself with the mother against the abusiveness and neglect of her husband. If the parents quarrel, it is most likely over the boy himself, or it may be over the functional inadequacies or cultural standards of one of the parents rather than over unsatisfactory sex relations which loomed large in the previous picture. The children too may quarrel constantly among themselves, but with little evidence of the consistent sibling rivalry and jealousy characteristic of both the unsocialized, aggressive child and the over-inhibited child.

The father's general indifference toward family responsibilities is further exemplified in his greater tendency to be lax in his methods of discipline and in his more openly expressed attitude of indifference toward this particular boy. It is the mother moreover who most frequently shields the boy from responsibility for his own acts. Both parents, however, may be extremely harsh in their attempts to secure discipline, using violent physical punishment and extreme measures of deprivation. The mother, in fact, may express a currently rejecting attitude toward her wayward son much as does the mother of the unsocialized, aggressive boy. It should be noted, however, that maternal rejection in this case is of comparatively recent origin and may presumably have developed in her despair over the trouble caused by her delinquent offspring. This child was not unwanted at birth, and whatever parental rejection developed shortly thereafter was displayed by the father rather than by the mother. Hence one should not be surprised to find this boy most resentful toward the father and, like the unsocialized, aggressive boy, feeling rejected by and hostile toward both parents. Once more the gross behavior may appear similar in both cases, but it arises from different circumstances and carries different implications.

Furthermore, the significant pressure in the family toward deviant behavior in this case would appear to come from the father rather than from the mother.

In brief, the boy showing a group delinquent reaction was typically given an adequate fundamental socialization in his relationship with his mother. Later, as a result of this socialization, the failure of paternal function, and the neighborhood deviation pressures, he fell under the influence of the delinquent gang and reached his adolescent socialization within a delinquent group.

Relation of Personality Structure to Culture

As a generalization, we are prepared to defend the following hypotheses:

A culture imposing little self-discipline is typically marked by a high incidence of overt external conflicts and a high incidence of primitive aggressive behavior. Competition for dominance is direct, undisguised, and primitive. The incidence of internal conflict and neuroticism is relatively low. As an example we would cite the lower-class American Negro community.

A culture imposing much self-discipline is typically marked by a low incidence of overt external conflicts and a low incidence of primitive aggressive behavior. Competition for dominance is canalized, disciplined, and often masked. The incidence of internal conflict and neuroticism is high. As an example we cite the American Jewish community.

As an instance related to differences in cultures, we would point out that women live under stronger social inhibitions than do men. It is therefore not surprising that they show a lower incidence of overt aggressive behavior, a competition for dominance which is more disguised and subtle, and a higher incidence of neuroticism.

Psychotherapy

The type of therapy needed is determined by the type of personality deviation with which we are dealing. First, let us consider the therapy of the over-inhibited, neurotic individual. This has been relatively well worked out. Indeed in the thinking of a vast number of people in psychiatry and mental hygiene the concept of psychiatric treatment is limited to the treatment appropriate for this particular type of problem, and to them nothing else is psychotherapy. With the first type of personality structure we are dealing with an individual in whom the shell of inhibition is too thick and too impenetrable. Obviously the treatment must be directed to canalize this shell of inhibition so that the primitive impulses may find some expression in a socially acceptable way. The manner in which this is done will depend upon the setting, but the same fundamental elements will be present whether one is dealing with an individual in a classroom relationship, in a foster home placement, or in intensive psychotherapy in the psychiatrist's office.

This method of therapy has been developed in its most elaborate form in the Freudian psychoanalysis. Here the therapist develops an essentially parental relationship to the patient. The parental nature of this relationship is recognized in the term which Freud applied to the patient's attitude toward his therapist —transfer. This expression is used because the patient's feeling for his therapist is recognized as a transfer of feelings which he previously had toward his parent. The psychoanalyst then proceeds to analyze the superego, essentially to take apart and canalize this shell of repression. To accomplish this purpose he puts his patient under a certain discipline—which is more or less parentally enforced. The requirement is that the patient shall freely associate, shall tell the therapist everything which comes into his mind. In this way the therapist is gradually able to bring the patient to relate those things of which he is conscious but of which he is ashamed. The therapist does not condemn the patient for these revelations, but is likely directly or indirectly to convey the impression that other people, too, think of such things, and to accept them as not shocking or unexpected. By the method of free association, by the interpretation of dreams, more and more of the unconscious repressed material is gradually brought to light. The patient may be shocked and distressed, but the therapist is not. He continues to accept the patient and, in this living therapeutic relationship, the patient gradually has the experience that here is a "parent" who does not reject him because of his secret nonconforming behavior or "evil" desires.

The therapist definitely leads the patient toward certain interpretations of his dreams and of his behavior. These interpretations are at least exceedingly likely to include a desire of the patient to violate the two most fundamental taboos of our culture—to kill his father and to have incestuous relations with his mother. We need not enter into the question of how frequently these interpretations may be justified. Interpretations do not *necessarily* have to be correct to be therapeutic, and one is not justified in arguing that an interpretation is necessarily correct because the patient accepts it with benefit. It should be apparent that when the patient has accepted such interpretations, and believes that he has these desires, and that his therapist believes that he has these desires and still does not reject him or regard him as wicked, then something has happened to reduce the insecurity responsible for his excessive shell of repression. The repression itself is not as tight and impenetrable as it was before. The primitive impulses can more readily find some overt and, we hope, not too unsocialized expression, and the inner conflict is in great part abated. The anxieties disappear and the neurotic symptoms are no longer needed to solve a conflict which is at least reduced in its intensity. The therapy is successful—at least to a degree. The patient improves.

This method of therapy is not adapted to the unsocialized, aggressive child. This point cannot be emphasized too strongly, as there is a widespread tendency to believe that if the analysis just goes deep enough a cure will inevitably result. Such a child as is represented in Type II does not have too much superego; he has too little. His behavior results not from inner conflict, but from a lack of it. One does not need to analyze a superego, rather it is necessary to synthesize one. One does not seek to relieve guilt-anxiety. One seeks to create it. This is done in essentially the way that taboos are planted at any time of life, whether in the early training period of childhood when the process is normally most intense or in later life readjustments as upon induction into the army. It requires the use of authority, firmness, planned limitation, and at times, punishment.

What is necessary for success is first of all a warm accepting attitude on the part of the parent or parent substitute. This is particularly important with the unsocialized, aggressive child who feels rejected and expects to be rejected. Until one has convinced such an individual of a fundamental interest in his welfare, therapy is not likely to be successful. It often requires an exceptional personality to be able to develop and maintain a high degree of personal warmth for some of these aggressive, unsocialized individuals whom most people are able to describe only in zoological metaphors.

Having established such a relationship, the next step is to establish and effectively maintain pressure toward required kinds of behavior and against certain objectionable types of behavior. This must be done step by step, often in very small steps. While an effort should be made to develop and exploit personal loyalty to one or more socialized adults, it must be recognized that this child's capacity for loyalty and identification is definitely feeble. The appeal must consequently be oriented in great part in terms of self-interest. Privileges which are abused must be withdrawn and returned step by step. For this reason older children and adolescents who are of the unsocialized, aggressive make-up usually cannot be effectively treated outside of an institution, because adequate control is impossible in the open democratically organized community. Constant reassurance of personal interest and warmth is necessary while particular patterns of behavior are disapproved. The reason that certain requirements are set upon the individual must be explained over and over again and the requirements must be made effective. Authoritative management and limitation which will be experienced and interpreted as punishment are essential portions of the treatment.

If one attempts to treat the unsocialized aggressive child by the methods suitable for the overinhibited, neurotic child, his behavior will typically get worse. Encouragement of the free expression of aggressiveness does not lead to improvement. An overinhibited person or a person of adequate inhibitions, who in a particular situation has developed special tension, may so relieve his feelings by a cathartic discharge of verbal hostilities, or acted out hostilities, as to be able to function effectively under the control only of his own conscience. This is not true of the child who lacks guilt feelings or any effective conscience. When treatment is undertaken by methods of play analysis, for example, if the therapist encourages more and more outpourings of the aggression, he will find that the well of hostility is bottomless. The therapeutic sessions may be made more frequent, but the hostile, aggressive, wild behavior only intensifies.

It must be recognized that the unsocialized, aggressive individual will frequently seek to protect himself from developing an attachment for anyone, and may respond negatively when he begins to feel himself becoming attached. This must be accepted as one of the problems of treatment.

As has been stated, treatment of the adolescent will usually need to be carried out in an institution, the major portion of it by someone who is in contact with the child much of the day. The social situation needs to be simplified by contact with fewer adults and with stable, mature, even-tempered and strong personalities. The maximum simplification should occur at the start, with a step-by-step increase in freedom and responsibility as the child is able to manage them. Psychotherapy has a place, but it is a very different type of psychotherapy than that employed with the overinhibited, neurotic, withdrawn individual. Psychotherapy here will be directed toward helping the patient recognize that his substitute parent is interested in his welfare, is not hostile, but is simply enforcing reasonable restrictions and that the wise course is to take advantage of the constructive opportunities the situation affords. This will have to be repeated over and over again and in different ways. There is an advantage in having a therapist not responsible (in the eyes of the child) for the authoritative decisions, participate or carry major responsibility for this psychotherapy. If this is criticized as superficial treatment, we would respond that it is as much of an error to use deep level therapy in a case requiring superficial treatment as it is to use only superficial treatment in a case which calls for deep level therapy.

The results of the treatment will be to develop somewhat the inadequate shell of inhibition, to stimulate foresight and an enlightened self-interest, and to develop certain patterns of conformity. If in addition skills are acquired, the prospect for an individual reasonably able to take his place in society may be good. In some extreme instances, only an improvement in the capacity for institutional adjustment may be realized.

The socialized delinquent or group delinquent boy (typically, this child is a boy) presents still another problem of treatment and one less "psychiatric" in that it is much closer to the ordinary techniques of influencing normal adults. This problem has been well discussed by Ruth Topping.[48] We are dealing with a child who had a fundamental socialization and then became a part of an aggressive minority group. He is a socialized person who resonates over too limited a scale. His fundamental socialization is expressed in his outstanding capacity for loyalty and this capacity, with the corresponding response to being given what he recognizes as a "break," plus his capacity to identify with and pattern himself after a masculine, socialized adult, are the major elements upon which one must depend.

The process of establishing rapport constitutes a major problem with the boy who is suspicious toward and well-armored against adults related in his mind to authority. If rapport is established, loyalty can be built by "giving him a break" or otherwise showing real interest and confidence in him. The circumstances should be such that he interprets the generous act or "break" as a result of personal interest and personal confidence, not as a result of weakness, fear, or an effort to "buy him off," for this boy typically despises weakness. The process of treatment then becomes a process of enlarging his concept of his in-group through the skillful development and utilization of his loyalty. Since he is part of a closely knit group, it is necessary for success effectively to separate him from this group, to neutralize its influence, or even as an alternative to treat the whole group. Particularly suited for work with this group are strong masculine personalities with capacity for warmth of response, generosity of feeling, utter fairness, and for uncompromising fixity of purpose. It should be delinquents of this group who would be most responsive to methods such as were employed by Clifford Shaw and his associates in the Area Projects in Chicago.

As a final comment, it is our hope that these considerations may stimulate the more discriminating thinking which is needed to resolve the conflicts between the educator often faced with the need to implant inhibitions, and the mental hygienist often faced with the need to reduce them.*

---

* Quoted from a study (by R. L. Jenkins and L. Hewitt) which appeared in the *American Journal of Orthopsychiatry*. Copyright, the American Orthopsychiatric Association, Inc. Reproduced by permission.

CHAPTER 5

ADJUSTMENT REACTIONS AND BEHAVIOR DISORDERS IN RELATION TO OTHER PSYCHIATRIC DIAGNOSES

To a considerable degree, human inadequacy in meeting the demands of life is a matter of becoming adjusted to a particular way of life, that is, to a particular set of demands and expectations. While there are obviously great differences in the capacities of different people to tolerate and adapt to change, still, it would appear that there is a limit to the tolerance of anyone. Those whose work faces them with frequent and profound changes often protect themselves by the careful cultivation of a daily routine in the limited portion of their lives that can be devoted to it.

We learn to cope with most of the problems which repeat themselves, and we spare ourselves some measure of strain by cultivating repetitive actions and repetitive solutions. We may find ourselves quite taken aback when there is a major change in our accustomed routine. Our accustomed solutions no longer work automatically and the resulting uncertainties may have a disturbing, or even a devastating effect upon us.

On the one hand, if there is too little variety in life, we may become bored. On the other, if there is too much, we may become insecure, or even confused. These generalizations apply to the developing child. If we take any child in a state of reasonable adaptation and make a large change in his daily life, we may destroy what has been, heretofore, an adequate or successful adjustment.

Indeed it is difficult in contemplating a change in the life

45

situation to realize how temporarily disruptive a loss of daily routine or even a major change in the daily routine may be. We may even underestimate the effect of a change in the inter-personal relationships in our lives. Changes in such important matters often cause some temporary disruption in our ways of coping with life.

Every child and every adolescent goes through various disturbing and even disrupting changes in life. Some youngsters are fortunate enough to have but few, and to be helped through them by understanding and supporting parents. Others have many, may not have supporting parents, or may lose their supporting parents in the process.

Those disturbing events which produce some transient disruption in the behavior or the intra-psychic processes, which seems to merit a diagnosis, are called *adjustment reactions.* Adjustment reactions are classified as *transient situational disturbances.* The diagnostician is asked to specify what has occasioned the reaction, and how it is expressed.

Of course it cannot be specified that a reaction is transient until it is over. If one were exacting about this, it would follow that an adjustment reaction could not be diagnosed as "adjustment reaction" until after it was over. That is, it could not be diagnosed an adjustment reaction except *in retrospect.* However, no one seems that rigid in the use of this diagnosis. As a consequence, what the diagnosis means in fact is that the diagnostician considers the behavior to be *reactive* and *expects it to be transient.*

There are many common causes for adjustment reactions in children. Perhaps the commonest is the birth of a younger sibling. That is not to imply that the birth of a younger sibling always, or even generally, causes an adjustment reaction in an older child. Quite the contrary. Most such transitions are accomplished without disturbing the mental health or the behavior of the older child to any important degree. However, disturbances in the older child are frequent at this time, particularly if the older child was heretofore an only child. Much depends upon whether or not the parents have been able to prepare the older child for the arrival of the younger one—and this in turn depends upon whether the age gap is enough for an explanation to be comprehended. Even more will depend upon whether, while the mother's attention is taken up with the new baby, the father, or others in the environment, take up the inevitable slack of the reduced maternal attention to the older child.

The possible causes of adjustment reactions are almost infinite. Common ones in addition to the birth of a new sibling are the illness or death of a parent, a divorce or the breakup of the home, the acquisition of a step-parent or step-siblings, gross or disturbing changes in living conditions or in school or in social relationships, such as are often involved in moving to a new neighborhood.

Some adjustment reactions are occasioned by reversible changes, such as the acute illness of the mother. In other cases the precipitating cause is irreversible, as the death of the mother. Nevertheless, over a period of time, most children adjust themselves to the loss of the mother *if* some adequate substitute parent takes her place. Such readjustment does not always occur. A child or adolescent who loses a parent and acquires in place an over critical and punitive step-parent may not readjust. Rather we may see the development of a repetitive pattern of running away from home to which we give the diagnostic label *runaway reaction.* This is a repetitive and, in the long run, a maladaptive type of response of trying to escape from a traumatic family situation.

The *runaway reaction* is one of the *behavior disorders of childhood and adolescence.* These disorders, while they usually begin as reactive disorders, become somewhat internalized as chronic maladaptive responses. They have a stability and a degree of internalization which are intermediate between the adjustment reactions and the personality disorders. If the feeling of rejection begins early enough and goes on long enough, we will ultimately see the basically unsocialized pattern of the *antisocial personality.*

It has been customary to distinguish the adjustment reactions by ages. In DSM-I the adjustment reactions of childhood, but *only* the adjustment reactions of childhood, were subdivided into conduct disturbance, habit disturbance and psychoneurotic traits. This particular subdivision was not called for with any other age group. In DSM-II this division has been dropped, but the diagnostician is asked to enter a statement of what the adjustment reaction is in response to, and what its symptomatic expression may be.

Finally DSM-II includes a new category of *social maladjustment without manifest psychiatric disorder*. Psychiatrists, as well as other professionals, often have brought to them problems of marital maladjustment. While occasionally such problems may be related to a diagnosable psychiatric disorder in one or even both of the marriage partners, usually they are not. The fact that two people who are married to each other do not get along together, can certainly not be interpreted to mean that either one is psychiatrically ill or disturbed, although marital maladjustment certainly *can* give rise to an adjustment reaction or even precipitate a more serious psychiatric disturbance.

In the same way we may see vocational maladjustment occur in a psychiatrically normal individual.

A third category is dyssocial behavior. This category should be reserved for those whose behavior is criminal or at least violates the rights of others, but who are otherwise psychiatrically normal. The reader may detect an inconsistency in that the *group delinquent reaction of adolescence* is accepted as a psychiatric diagnosis, a behavior disorder, while the same behavior in adult life will be classified as *social maladjustment without manifest psychiatric disorder, dyssocial behavior*. However, this inconsistency is predicated upon society's present tendency, in considering adult offenses, to draw a sharper line between psychiatric illness and delinquent behavior than it does in its present practice with children and adolescents.

CHAPTER 6

THE OVERANXIOUS REACTION
(The Conflicted Worrier)

MAN IS NOT HAPPY IN ISOLATION. IN GENERAL HE IS MOST UN-
HAPPY TO EXPERIENCE THE DISAPPROVAL OF HIS FELLOWS, ALTHOUGH
THIS DISAPPROVAL MAY BE TOLERATED VERY WELL IF HE IS SUSTAINED
BY THE APPROVAL OF A SMALL IN-GROUP. HE BECOMES AN ADULT
HUMAN THROUGH A LONG PROCESS OF SOCIALIZATION. THIS IS A
PROCESS OF ACCEPTING OR ADAPTING TO THE STANDARDS AND VALUES
OF HIS FELLOWS.

It is the mother person, first of all, who is important to the
child. He begins to respond emotionally and feel secure as her
ministrations meet his needs. Sigmund Freud emphasized the
importance of oral satisfactions in the early affectionate responses
of the child. While feeding is necessary to survive, it now seems
highly probable that the sensory stimulation involved in holding
and rocking is even more central to the development of social
response. It has been demonstrated that holding and rocking
with aural stimulation such as speech or cooing definitely increases vocal responses and social responsiveness of young infants
so treated over control infants in a rather short span of time.[38]

During the latter part of infancy, there is definitely social
interaction between mother and child. The infant learns that
some actions and responses bring maternal approval, while others
do not. As speech gradually develops in the child, he learns
increasingly the value, positive or negative, that his mother puts
on various of his actions. He now has two motivational drives,
one innate and a response initially of his own nature, and the
other acquired from the actions and value system of his mother.

Not infrequently these two motivations will pull him in opposite and sometimes irreconcilable directions. This is the beginning of a state of inner conflict.

It is not possible to have social living without inner conflict. A tyrant, adult, or child, may temporarily succeed in imposing his will upon others, without suffering inner conflict himself, but in so doing he necessarily increases the inner conflict of those about him.

Having recognized that inner conflict is invariably a part of social living, we may consider elements that increase it or diminish it. These should be related to psychoneurosis in adults and, in children, to psychoneurosis or to what has been called in these pages *the overanxious reaction*. We note the following elements:

1. Parental warmth and the security of the child in the home will diminish the tendency toward anxiety. By the same token, the failure of parents to make a child feel secure for *who he is*— a member of the family—is anxiety-provoking. The explicit or implied requirement that his recognition and approval as a member of the family is dependent upon his good behavior or good performance provokes further anxiety, particularly in the child who lacks confidence in himself. Encouragement toward a good level of achievement does not require the creation of insecurity. However, ambitious families often create in their children anxiety over achievement, to a degree which may be devastating in its effect.

2. The child's own level of self-confidence is important. In this the child of good abilities is in a much more favorable situation than the child who has difficulties in keeping up with other children. Much childhood illness, or special disabilities in the child render him more vulnerable to anxiety.

3. Anxiety in the parent renders the child more vulnerable, for anxiety is easily communicated, particularly from a mother to a dependent child.

4. The child's view of the world as a threatening and hostile place, or as a more friendly and perhaps manageable environment, is significant. A belief in the possibility of some constructive synthesis of potentially conflicting demands may be anxiety-

reducing. Thus the child made anxious by strong parental demands for scholarship may tolerate these well if he is able to relate constructively on a personal level with his teacher, or if he is able to find some personal interest or gratification in what he learns through his studies.

Here is one example of anxiety resulting from early emotional deprivation:

> Helen was 14 when referred to a state mental hospital by a local psychiatrist after she had been hospitalized on the psychiatric ward of a general hospital six or seven times.
>
> Helen was the second of three children, with an older brother and a younger brother three years her junior.
>
> The marriage of her parents was always a conflicted and rocky one. The mother gave in to the needs of her husband until she had a nervous breakdown when Helen was 12 years of age. Then the parents were divorced. The youngest boy remained with the mother but Helen and her older brother shuttled back and forth between the homes of their father and their mother.
>
> Helen was a shy girl who did not like to argue or fight. She grew up in a rough neighborhood and began to be withdrawn in the first or second grade in school. Her problem intensified and by 5th grade she was almost friendless in her own age group. She had great difficulty in expressing her feelings. Helen's father was critical of her and unsympathetic, and both parents involved the children in their conflict with each other. Helen began to experiment with drugs and had some bad trips. Treatment was undertaken through a community mental health center.
>
> When Helen became upset, she would become withdrawn, talk much of suicide or threaten suicide and would be taken to the hospital. On her last hospitalization on the psychiatric ward, she refused to leave when the doctor was ready to discharge her, because she did not want to live with either parent, and she welcomed her transfer to a state mental hospital as an alternative. The diagnosis of the referring psychiatrist was **schizophrenia,** complicated by family problems and drug usage.
>
> In the hospital, Helen tested in the average range in intelligence. The psychologist felt that Helen was trying to control

intense anger which she felt, by isolating herself. Her social skills were poorly developed.

The psychiatrist felt that Helen's anger was primarily self-directed. He was impressed with her generally depressed attitude and mood relating to her home situation. His diagnosis was **overanxious reaction of adolescence.**

In the hospital, Helen initially had half hour sessions of psychotherapy daily and responded rather well to these. She became fearful that her father would sell her horse. She was much attached to the horse and visited it when she had the opportunity. In psychotherapy, she talked much in metaphor about her horse and her dog and their feelings of rejection. Her horse presumably was stolen. Its whereabouts were known, but the father refused to reclaim it. Her dog remained with her mother.

Despite good features and very attractive coloring, Helen felt that she was not pretty and, of course, she lacked self-confidence. Initially, she was quite aloof in school. She would do her assigned work carefully and accurately but would not inform the teacher when it was complete. Her schoolwork steadily improved and she gradually gained some measure of confidence.

Helen's mother showed a dependable interest with regular visits and a cooperative attitude. She began home visits to her mother's home.

At present, Helen has been in the hospital ten months. She has had ten visits to her mother's home; they have gone well. She is doing well in school. She was elected chairman of the adolescent ward government and managed that office quietly but judiciously and well. While she is still insecure, she has good assets and has become more aware of them. We regard the prognosis as favorable and the diagnosis of schizophrenia as incorrect.*

The vast majority of overanxious children can be managed successfully in their homes if the parents are willing to cooperate in the treatment. The foregoing case is an unusually severe one.

------

* Helen was released from the hospital about a month after this abstract was completed and is living with her mother. Reportedly she is making a rather good adjustment. She is back in school and is showing a less passive attitude than in her earlier school experience. We regard the prognosis as quite favorable.

In 1946 a paper by Sylvia Glickman and myself[25] noted what we then called the overinhibited child as comprising one of the three best-defined clusters of inter-correlated traits in Ackerson's study[1] of 5,000 children examined at the Institute for Juvenile Research. Among 2,113 boys aged 6 to 16 years inclusive, with an IQ of 50 or above, who were or had been in the public schools, this is what we found. The central traits of this cluster were: *sensitiveness over some specific fact or episode;* the staff notation of *inferiority feelings; depressed or discouraged attitude or spells of depression or discouragement; worry over some specific fact or episode;* the staff notation of *mental conflict; unhappy or discontented attitude, appearance, or manner;* the staff notation of *psychoneurotic trends; sensitiveness* (as a general trait); *seclusiveness* and *daydreaming.*

In a similar population of 1,118 girls, the central traits were a staff notation of *inferiority feelings, depressed or discouraged attitude,* or *spells of depression or discouragement, sensitiveness, sensitiveness over some specific fact or episode, daydreaming, crying spells* or *crying easily,* and *seclusiveness.*

A reworking of the Michigan Child Guidance Institute data by computer clustering[12] resulted in two clusters bearing some relation to the foregoing—one a shy-seclusive group which relates with the *withdrawing reaction,* and the other an overanxious-neurotic group which relates to the *overanxious reaction.* The 43 children in this latter group had at least 3 of the traits *sleep disturbance, fears, cries easily, fantastic thinking* (overimaginative), *marked inferiority feeling* and *nervousness.* Thirty-seven per cent were girls and the interquantile range was 9 to 12. As we compared these children with those in the shy-seclusive group, they more typically showed a higher level of parental education and an overanxious but otherwise competent mother. Most of these children had a history of prolonged serious or repeated illness, and a substantial incidence of restless hyperactivity.

Hilda Lewis,[32] in seeking to verify our findings, defined constraint as child management involving at least two of the following:

1. Rigid daily program.
2. Excessive discipline by parent or in children's home or residential school.
3. Domination and hyper-criticism by parent.
4. Lack of warmth within family or group.
5. Enforced isolation or social ostracism.
6. Over-protection.

Dr. Lewis found this pattern of management significantly more frequent in her inhibited-neurotic group than in the children she classified as socialized delinquent or as unsocialized aggressive.

From the 1,500 IJR cases,[14, 15] 287 children were selected for the presence of at least two of these entries: *chronically anxious and fearful, shy, generally immature, reluctance to attend or fear of school, overly conforming, submissive, difficulty in separating from the mother, frequent nightmares,* and *sleep disturbance other than nightmares.*

Our group of 287 children classified as overanxious included 139 (or 74 per cent) of 188 children described as *chronically anxious and fearful.* The other 49 children were not included as they showed none of the other entries. Our overanxious group included 107 (74 per cent) of 144 children described as *shy.* It included 45 (68 per cent) of 66 children showing *difficulty in separating from mother* for the psychiatric examinations, 56 (65 per cent) of 86 children described as *overly conforming, submissive,* 45 (64 per cent) of 70 children afflicted with *sleep disturbances other than nightmares* and 49 (62 per cent) of 79 with *frequent nightmares.* It included 90 (54 per cent) of 167 children showing *reluctance to attend or fear of school* and 189 (47 per cent) of 402 children described as *generally immature.*

Although a majority of overanxious children in the IJR material are males (about 2 out of 3), this is a very significantly lower proportion ($p < .001$) than that for the remainder of the children (about 4 out of 5).

Ages under 8 years were slightly over-represented compared with the clinic population in general. Small families were over-represented, particularly the two-child family.

The source of referral was preponderantly medical and was more likely to be medical than for clinic children in general.

From the social history, the patient was the product of a planned pregnancy significantly more frequently than was the case for clinic children in general. In a disproportional number of cases the child was described as in poor condition at delivery. This was probably a factor contributing to parental and particularly to maternal anxiety.

Difficulties in speech are less frequent than the clinic average. Infantile speech is the only characteristic difficulty.

In response to inquiry about methods of discipline, the parent was very unlikely to describe withdrawal of privileges as a method of discipline. They were also unlikely (compared with the clinic average) to describe *physical punishment* as a method of discipline. In general these anxious children probably needed little discipline to control their behavior.

With more than chance frequency, these children had a bed alone in their parents' bedroom.

Marital conflict is less frequent in their homes than is the clinic average. When it does occur, the reasons the parents give for conflict between them are unlikely to be economic but are likely to be personality differences.

The patient is unlikely to be characterized as *usually a leader.*

The social worker is quite likely to characterize the mother's attitude toward the child as *infantilizing, overprotective.*

The psychologist found the number of children who fall in the *superior, very superior* range significantly below the clinic average. The test findings were seriously questioned by the psychologist more frequently than in the average clinic case.

The psychologist typically described the child's relationship with him as *shy, withdrawn, inhibited,* or as *ill at ease, apprehensive.* The child's relationship with his environment was described as *withdrawn, passive* and the manifestation of hostility was described as *minimal, hostility repressed.* The child's relationship with his parents as estimated by the psychologist, was *submissive.*

The psychiatric examination listed, as compared with the

average clinic child, an absence of such overt behavior as *stealing* and *lying. Bullying, domineering, aggressive* was generally omitted as a personality difficulty. However, these children were selectively checked for the personality difficulties interfering with peer relations: *withdrawn, seclusive, daydreaming,* and *victimized, teased.* They were also prone to be rated as *depressed, discouraged;* and enuresis as a regressive phenomenon (that is, its reappearance after toilet training had been established) was very prominent. At the .05 level of significance, *nail biting* also appears.

The psychiatrist typically classified the primary problem area as *personality difficulties,* and specifically not as *socially unacceptable acts.* The relationship made by the child with the psychiatrist was most often described as *ill at ease, apprehensive* or as *passive with superficial compliance.* Occasionally it was described as *suspicious, uncommunicative.* A special feature highly characteristic of the interview was the *general immaturity* of the patient. Sometimes the child was checked as *noticeably depressed.*

The items typically checked in the psychiatrist's estimate of the mother's relation with the child were an *infantilizing, overprotective* relationship by the mother and the mother's *setting example for child's pathology.* A *marked preference for patient* on the part of the mother and maternal *lack of consistency* were also checked.

Paternal factors are infrequent and appear relatively unimportant compared with maternal factors in these cases. The most prominent factor is *paternal irresponsibility, poor work record* which doubtless relates to the item often checked under parental relationship, *partner frequently absent from the home.* The entry marked *overt parent conflict* is less frequent than in the clinic population in general.

Under the parents concept of self-involvement in the patient's problem, *maternal ambivalence* is frequently checked.

The whole picture is one of the timid child who has been taught to rely on the strength of others in a dependent relationship and who has learned this lesson too well. By implication we get as occasional contributing factors the picture of an over-anxious mother who may have been frightened by delivering a planned child which proved in poor condition at birth and who is likely to have had little emotional support and perhaps even little material support from her husband.

In the intake information study of 300 cases in Iowa City,[28] we compared 172 children definitely classed as overanxious, over-conforming, with 128 not so classified. This, of course, is more than half of our cases.

These children were typically referred for neurotic traits and/or physical symptoms which did not develop until after six years of age.

Their parents selectively checked *sensitive* as a descriptive adjective and selectively avoid checking *doesn't care, untruthful* and *won't mind.* This would imply that these children were seen by their parents as concerned, truthful and obedient as well as sensitive beyond the clinic average.

These children attended school, were unlikely to present behavior problems, and the parents typically believed that the school understood the child.

The child's early development was reported to be normal, and the child was unlikely to be reported as having colic in his first six months.

This child's family was typically stable and the child was living with both parents. The father was more than usually likely to be of the professional-managerial occupation group. However, this group contained more than its quota of adopted children, presumably because it is mostly middle class families that adopt children. Both parents reported their relation to the child to involve more harmony than conflict. The mother typically feels partially responsible for the conflict. Both parents, but particularly the mother, are more than usually likely to wish a college education for the child. The parents were likely to report that they relied particularly on discussion for disciplinary control.

In these cases the clinic recommendations were most likely to be carried out. Müller and Shamsie[34] in applying my original grouping in an electroencephalographic study of 78 teenager girls on the Adolescent Service of the Douglas Hospital in Montreal, found that the "overinhibited" teenage girls "showed more fast activity in temporal areas, a stronger reaction to eye opening and more positive spikes during chlorpromazine-induced sleep than the others." This certainly suggests a contributory physiological factor.

With the overanxious child in the clinic, treatment begins with supportive treatment and may proceed to interpretation and the giving of insight if and when the patient is ready for such treatment. The central elements of treatment of the overanxious child, however, are to work with parents to help them understand and learn how to meet the child's need for parental acceptance and support in a way which he does not feel to be conditional on his good performance.

CHAPTER 7

THE UNSOCIALIZED AGGRESSIVE REACTION

(The Fighting Response)

MAN IS A SOCIAL ANIMAL—BUT HE LIKES HIS OWN WAY! THE CAPACITY TO GIVE UP ONE'S IMMEDIATE AND SELFISH DESIRES FOR THE RIGHTS OR DESIRES OF OTHERS IS ACQUIRED ONLY UNDER FAVORABLE CIRCUMSTANCES AND BY LONG DISCIPLINE. ITS DEVELOPMENT CALLS FOR EMPATHY WITH OTHERS, AND THIS DEPENDS, MORE THAN ON ANYTHING ELSE, ON A WARM CONFIDENT RELATION WITH A PARENT-PERSON, USUALLY A MOTHER, BEGINNING VERY EARLY IN LIFE. THE RAPPORT WHICH BEGINS WITH A SUCCESSFUL PARENT-CHILD AND CHILD-PARENT RELATIONSHIP IS THE ANLAGE OF THE CAPACITY FOR SUCCESSFUL INTERPERSONAL RAPPORT. MORALITY BEGINS WITH LOYALTY, USUALLY TO A PARENT-PERSON, AND THE DESIRE TO PLEASE THAT PARENT-PERSON THROUGH ONE'S BEHAVIOR AND THROUGH ACCEPTANCE OF THAT PERSON'S STANDARDS OF BEHAVIOR.

Which of us has not wanted to scream defiance at some social demand, to retaliate against or attack the person making a demand we felt to be unreasonable? Most of us have not only felt this way; most of us have at some time acted this way in our younger years. But most of us, as children, get over and give up this kind of behavior. We do so more readily if we feel that the established system of social organization gives us some measure of protection with regard to rights that are ours, as well as denying us things we desire which rightfully belong to someone else. Indeed, we learn to respect the rights of others most easily if we admire and pattern ourselves after some older person who himself respects those rights and the law. Furthermore we learn such conformity more readily if the rules appear reasonable and are applied consistently. We learn it most easily if the law and the rules *protect,* as well as limit us.

The following case gives a clear instance of the unsocialized, aggressive reaction one can expect from a child with (possibly) hyperkinetic tendencies in a home without effective parenting. Here successful interpersonal rapport never does occur or is long delayed.

Phillip was an illegitimate child. His mother was a senior in high school living at home when she became pregnant. Her parents were reported to be extremely angry about this, and to have insisted that she keep the baby and help raise it.

Phillip was reported to be "three months premature," to have had a birth weight of 5 lb. 9 oz., to have been a blue baby, and to have been left in oxygen for 24 hours.

Phillip's mother was in school and most of the burden of his care fell upon his grandmother. Phillip's mother ran off with a man, married him and had a second child. The marriage broke up and she left this child with its father. She had three more pregnancies and carried one to term. This child was placed in adoption. She married again, had a child and was divorced. At last information she was living with her third husband and their four children.

Phillip's toilet training was not successful and he remained a bedwetter for some years. At the age of five years his maternal grandparents, who had raised him, adopted him when they became concerned that his mother might claim him. He showed anxiety at separation from his adoptive mother when he began school. He was then in a serious car accident, fatal to one person in the other car, in which his adoptive mother was injured. Phillip did not appear to be injured but was troubled with a slight transient memory loss, probably a direct, immediate result of the impact. Subesquently, he suffered from nightmares, fear of the dark, and an exacerbation of his fear of separation from his mother. In any event, this accident affected his adoptive family adversely. Phillip was not responsive to his adoptive father, and this man largely gave up his efforts with Phillip.

Phillip's school progress was not very good. According to his own account, he could not stay in his seat in first grade. He repeated third grade and then was in a special room for under-achievers. At 11 years of age, he was examined by a psychologist in a field clinic for crippled children. This psychologist was impressed with Phillip's tendency to see his adoptive father as a threatening, potentially destructive individual and by the repetitive-ness of his tending to blame others for his problem of adjustment. A lack of impulse control was very evident at this time.

When Phillip was 12 an examination was arranged in the out-patient department of a state mental hospital. This indicated average intelligence but a school achievement of 3rd and low 4th grade level at 12 years of age. The school principal's comment on Phillip's behavior was as follows:

> This child has been a continual problem since coming to our school. He does not get along on the playground because he is mean to other children. He disobeys school rules, sasses the patrol children, and defies all authority.
>
> He has been suspended from cafeteria privileges several times for fighting, pushing, and shoving. After misbehaving one day at the cafeteria, the teacher told him to come up to my office to see me. He flatly refused, laid on the floor, and threw a temper tantrum by kicking and screaming.
>
> The truth is not in Phillip. When caught in actual acts of misdeeds, he will deny it, and he takes upon himself the air of injured innocence. He believes we are picking on him. His attitude is sullen when he is refused anything. He pouts and sasses.
>
> Phillip is very aggressive on the bus and has had trouble with others while riding home and while coming to school. When asked why he does a certain thing, he points to his head and says, "Because I'm not right up here."
>
> This boy needs help badly. He does not seem to have friends. His aggressive behavior prevents the children from liking him.

Phillip's examination underlines the problems of his inability to concentrate, his low tolerance for frustration, his aggressive behavior and poor impulse control, his restlessness and instability. He saw his parents as strict and punitive and as having little concern for him, and indeed the outstanding characteristics of the home for him seemed to be rejection and rigidity.

The diagnosis at this time was adjustment reaction of child-hood, conduct disorder. Suggestions were made to the school for working with his parents. Phillip was placed on some mild tran-quilizers and a three month return appointment was arranged. However, before this date arrived he was excluded from school, after two suspensions for uncontrollability. He was then admitted to the children's unit then available in a state mental hospital in his state.

At first he showed marked difficulties in all areas of the pro-gram. Gradually he became a little more mature, more cooperative and more willing to accept limits on his behavior. Meanwhile work with his adoptive parents helped them see that they had been over-protective and had not been able to set firm and consistent limits. They were, however, quite elderly and not strong. After eight months Phillip was discharged as having received maximal hospital benefit with a statement that the prognosis was not favorable. Close contact with Phillip had been preserved with Phillip's school psychologist during this hospitalization and he returned to public school in his small community.

Over the next two years Phillip's behavior gradually deteriorated, with much involvement in name-calling, fights, and refusal to obey school personnel. He was suspended following the discovery in his locker of a tape recorder missing from a school office. Phillip denied having taken the recorder, but he had put on his locker an extra special padlock which he brought from home.

At this time the adoptive parents recognized that they could no longer cope with Phillip and accepted his commitment to the mental hospital. At age 14 Phillip was admitted to the adolescent unit of a nearby state mental hospital on a juvenile court petition as a dependent child in need of special care and treatment his parents were unable to provide.

Phillip's course in the hospital was an extremely stormy one. He made himself unpopular with his peers by repeatedly stealing from them. When confronted with this he would lie or refuse to answer. He was hostile and uncooperative and when crossed he would become combative in an all-out manner which was controlled only with difficulty and at the expense of barked shins etc. He was particularly inclined to a foul mouth and to use derogatory, insulting language. As a result of his behavior he spent much time in seclusion, but he was very slow to learn to modify his behavior at all. While in seclusion he destroyed his mattress by cutting it with a piece of glass. He was expected to work off the cost.

Projective tests made it clear that Phillip saw himself as mistreated by a hostile world and that he had a very poor self-image.

His restlessness, impulsiveness and short attention span were so gross as to excite frequent staff comment. An EEG was abnormal with 14 and 6 per second positive spike discharges on the left during drowsiness, and with 3 to 5 slow waves showing up during hyperventilation with a slow recovery.

When Phillip went out of control, he seemed to go out of control completely and communication became impossible until after he was overpowered and had time to cool down.

His relation with staff began to improve as they persisted in showing interest and goodwill in spite of his assaultiveness. His relations with his peer group improved much more slowly.

Elements which seemed to help keep Phillip motivated were a good singing voice, for which he received some recogintion, and visits from his adoptive parents, who saw him making slow progress in the hospital and who would occasionally visit and take him out to dinner. Although they could not control him themselves, they did cooperate with the hospital.

Real progress began when he was assigned to work with some of the maintenance staff. He took to this work and intermittently he performed well on it.

There were apparently two significant factors contributing to Phillip's problem. The description of his early behavior is that of a child showing a *hyperkinetic reaction,* as will be described in a later chapter (Chapter 12). He was premature, was described as a blue baby, and was put in oxygen. There is good reason to suspect that he suffered some slight brain damage from anoxia at birth. The EEG supports this suspicion, as of course does the hyperkinetic syndrome.

Phillip, a child we suspect was handicapped by minimal brain damage, was not warmly received in his home. His mother's parents insisted that she keep him, apparently feeling that she deserved this. She turned the tables on them by running away with a man, leaving them to take care of her first child. Her second child she left with her first ex-husband and her third child she placed in adoption. Phillip's grandparents adopted Phillip when they feared that their daughter might claim him. Phillip's adoptive parents had not had much success in training their own children.

As a youngster handicapped by restlessness, distractibility, short attention span and impulsiveness Phillip lived in what he felt to be a hostile world, but one which typically gave ground under his attack. Phillip's grandfather was critical and rigid, but gave up with Phillip. His grandmother was emotional but inconsistent and ineffective in controlling Phillip. Phillip's pattern of attack often brought him the immediate results he wanted, and Phillip came to the hospital with much to unlearn. It is our hope that Phillip's present interest in work will make it possible for him to make an adjustment in the community.*

In the clustering of Ackerson's data,[1, 25] the unsocialized aggressive child formed one of the three best-defined clusters. Among 2,113 boys 6 to 18 years of age inclusive, of IQ 50 and above, who were or had been in the public schools, the central traits in the cluster were *disturbing influence in school, fighting, quarrelsomeness, destructiveness, incorrigibility, boastfulness, teasing other children, exclusion from school* and *unpopularity.* In a similar population of 1,118 girls, the central traits of the cluster were *violence, fighting, incorrigibility, temper tantrums, defiant attitude, disobedience, disturbing influence in school, rudeness, quarrelsomeness, exclusion from school, lying, unpopularity, leading others into bad conduct, destructiveness,* and *queerness.*

---

* Shortly after this abstract was prepared, Phillip was transferred from the adolescent ward to a closed adult men's ward. Here his combativeness rapidly diminished and his adjustment accordingly approved. Phillip ascribed this improvement to the fact that he was no longer in contact with other poorly controlled adolescents who tended to stir him up and provoke him. After about three months he was returned to the home of his adoptive parents and presently (six weeks later) is making a satisfactory adjustment. He attends school mornings and works in a gas station in the afternoons in a school-work program. We regard the prognosis as presently favorable.

In Japan, a study by Kobayashi, Mizushima, and Shinohara[30] of 200 boys 6 to 15 years of age, yielded four clusters of inter-correlated traits of which one gave the traits of the unsocialized aggressive group. The "primary" or central traits were *quarrelsomeness, bravado, rudeness toward persons in authority, starting fights, malicious mischief,* and *defiance of authority. Mischievousness* was listed as a "secondary symptom," and "peripheral symptoms" included *emotional outbursts, assaultive tendencies, bossiness, cruelty, negativism, obscene and profane language, smoking, projection of blame,* and *unkindness.*

A reworking of the MGGI data by computer[12] revealed the existence in this clinic population of an "undomesticated" group of children characterized by *negativism, defiance of authority, vengefulness, sullenness, malicious mischief,* and *temper outbursts.* This cluster again focuses on the unsocialized aggressive. There were 58 children among the 500 who had at least 3 of these traits and also had more traits in this group than in any other. Seventy-six per cent were boys and the interquantile age range was 11 to 14. This research underlined the disproportionate frequency of maternal rejection in infancy experienced by these children (55 per cent), the unstable mother unable to relate herself to responsibility (38 per cent), the frequency with which the child was openly hostile to the natural mother (24 per cent), and the rarity with which the child preferred the natural mother to the other parent or parents (2 per cent).

The late Hilda Lewis of London, using rather stringent criteria,[32] found 52 unsocialized aggressive children among 500 followed up from the Mersham Reception Center and found lack of maternal affection, lack of paternal affection, being in public care before placement at Mersham, and illegitimacy all associated with the unsocialized aggressive pattern of behavior. Parental rejection, carefully defined, was associated with the unsocialized aggressive reaction at the .001 level of significance.

A computer study[14, 15] was undertaken of 1,500 cases examined and coded at the Illinois Institute for Juvenile Research. The selection of unsocialized aggressive children was made in terms of the presence of at least two of six behavioral entries: *destructiveness, lying, firesetting, disobedience with a hostile component, temper,* and personality difficulties described as *bullying, domineering, aggressive.*

This group included 134 (84 per cent) of 159 children with the entry of *destructiveness,* 191 (84 per cent) of 227 children listed with *lying* as a problem, and 54 (77 per cent) of 70 children with the entry *firesetting.* It includes 232 (74 per cent) of 314 with the entry *temper,* and 220 (56 per cent) of 396 children described as *bullying, domineering, aggressive.*

Eighty per cent of these children were boys, a percentage significantly higher than the clinic average of 74 per cent. It is decidedly less common for both natural parents of these children to be in the home than with the average clinic child. These parents were characteristically separated or divorced, and the missing parent, most often the father, might be replaced by a step-parent. Having middle position in a sibship of three or four children seemed to be a slightly predisposing factor. Youngest children are under-represented. That is to say, there is an over-representation of those birth positions in which maternal attention is likely to be relatively lacking, and an under-representation of the birth position where it is likely to be more abundant.

Referral was typically suggested by a school, not by a medical source. In parental occupations, the upper managerial group was under-represented, while service workers were over-represented. The economic status of the family was a little less likely to be adequate for these children than for the average child seen in the clinic.

The pregnancy was reported to have been planned in only one case out of five, a frequency significantly below the clinic average. It is of interest that half of the cases in which the parents reported an attempted abortion fell in this group. This report is 2½ times as frequent in this group as in the remaining cases, although, with the small numbers involved, it meets only the 0.1 level of significance (two tailed distribution) and consequently is below our selected limit of significance. Had the direction of the expected deviation been specified in advance (it was not) a one-tailed distribution might properly have been used and this would have given a .05 level of significance.

Fewer of these children were reported by their mothers to

be unusually quiet (inactive) in infancy than was the case with the remaining clinic population.

The mother was unlikely to have been relaxed about toilet training.

A small but significantly higher fraction of these children than of the clinic population in general shared a bed with a sibling of the opposite sex.

Methods of discipline reported more frequently by the parents of these children than by the parents of the remaining children include *physical punishment, withdrawal of privileges, physical restraint or confinement, physical or emotional isolation* and *bribery.*

The mother's attitude toward this child, as recorded by the social worker, was with significant frequency one of *overt rejection,* was *critical, depreciative, lacking consistency,* was *punitive* or involved *acting out through the child.* This last implied that in the judgment of the social worker the mother was encouraging the child's delinquent behavior by her own enjoyment of it or motivation toward it. Such encouragement is usually unconscious. Compared with the mothers of the remaining cases, these mothers were likely to report a problem of alcoholism in the household in which they grew up.

The father's attitude was seen by the social worker as frequently *lacking consistency* and as not likely to be judged *reasonably wholesome.*

The relationship of the child with the psychologist tended to be *provocative* and was unlikely to be described as *shy, withdrawn, or inhibited.* The psychologist described the child's manifestation of hostility as *excessive, easily elicited,* his relationship with the environment as *acting out,* not as *withdrawn-passive.* The child's relation with his parents was *hostile-aggressive.* The child's attitude (interest, motivation) in relation to the tests was not likely to be described as *focused, sustained, goal-directed.* The psychologists' estimate of a good prognosis in treatment was less than usually frequent.

Aside from those on which this group was selected, the socially unacceptable acts characterizing this group were *disobedience,* in general, *solitary stealing, truancy from school* and *running away from home. Excessive sexual interest* was common. These children tended to be *overly competitive with siblings* and *overly competitive with other children.* They were *restless, excitable.* A failure of toilet training in the form of a persistent *enuresis* was more than usually common, as was a *feeding problem.*

In the psychiatrist's opinion the primary problem area was *socially unacceptable acts* and the problem was *frequent or constant.* The psychiatrist was unlikely to record that there were *few personality deviations.*

The relation made by the psychiatrist with the child was likely to be poor, either *overanimated, uninhibited,* or *guarded, defensive, resistive.* In the interview there was likely to be *motor restlessness or incoordination.* Often the psychiatrist noted *play or fantasy poorly organized* and that the child might be *noticeably depressed.* The psychiatrst's impression was likely to be that the child was *severely disturbed.*

Dynamic factors in the home noted by the psychiatrist in order of their prominence were *more than one placement in the past, acquisition of a new sibling or parent, loss of a parent (or parents), both parents working,* and *marked economic problems.* Both the father and the mother were less likely to be *reasonably concerned* with the problem than the parents of other clinic children.

In the judgment of the psychiatrist in these cases neither parent is likely to have a *reasonably wholesome* attitude toward the child. The mother is rated as *punitive,* as *lacking consistency,* as *overly permissive,* as showing *overt rejection,* being *critical, depreciative,* being *cold, distant, neglectful,* as *conflicting with other authorities* (usually the father), as *delegating parental responsibility to others,* and sometimes as *rivalrous* with the child. She was not described as *infantilizing, overprotective,* nor as *overly ambitious* as often as were the mothers of the remaining children. The father was rated as *punitive, lacking consistency, conflicting with other authorities,* being *overly permissive* and *rivalrous* with the child. The rating of *rivalrous* with the child, which appears with a significantly elevated frequency with both parents, reflects their emotional immaturity. Parents whose own needs for acceptance and emotional dependency have never been met are likely to show such rivalry.

With these parents the psychiatrist is both unlikely and less than usually likely to consider either parent as *within or close to normal limits*. His recording on the mother is usually *character disturbance or psychoneurosis*. With the father it is likely to be *alcoholism, delinquency* or *irresponsibility, poor work record*.

The parental relationship is unlikely to rate as *reasonably satisfactory*. *Marked depreciation of marital partner* is very common. The *stepmother* and *stepfather* in the home are both very frequent.

The parents bringing children to the Child Psychiatry Service at the University of Iowa are asked to fill out an intake questionnaire. We collected 300 cases in which this had been done.[28] We classified 48 of these 300 as showing a definite pattern of unsocialized-aggressive or poorly socialized behavior. We then compared these 48 cases with the remaining 252 cases not so classified.

Referral of the unsocialized aggressive children was typically occasioned by a specific event of destructiveness or overaggressive behavior. Referral was likely to be by a juvenile court and was less than usually likely to be from a physician.

On a checklist of adjective and descriptive phrases the parents of these children checked items to describe their children as *cruel, resents authority, doesn't care, inconsiderate, untruthful, resentful, inadequate* and *won't mind*. According to the parents, these children are disposed to hide, break and destroy things, and more than a proportionate number have run away from home.

In relation to sleep habits the parents check the child's bedtime as *irregular* and the sleep difficulty as *cannot go to sleep*.

Typically the child had been truant from school and had been a behavior problem at school. The parents did not feel that the school understood the child.

The child's birth was not the result of a planned pregnancy. However, the mother was less likely than the average mother to report that she suffered from nausea and vomiting during pregnancy. Nighttime bladder training was likely not to have been achieved at 37 months.

The outstanding family characteristic was the great frequency and degree of family instability. The child's parents were likely not to be living together. With a disproportionate frequency the child was raised in part by a stepparent or even not raised by either parent. Both parents were likely to have had more than one marriage before the birth of the child and both were likely to have remarried since the birth of the child. The father was likely to report that the father-child relationship involved more conflict than harmony. The father was likely to feel that the mother did not understand the problem as well as he did, and the mother was not likely to feel herself partially to blame for the child's problem. Neither parent aspired to the child's going beyond high school.

The total picture is that of the unplanned and often unwanted child, born to emotionally immature parents who are punitive, inconsistent and overly permissive, who are likely to be rivalrous with the child and who have a notably unstable relationship with each other. In such a home it is not surprising that a child grows up unsocialized. When, with this background, a child grows up with a good musculature, he is likely to be aggressive if he dares to be. If, in addition to their own aggressive behavior toward him, his parents shield him from authorities and from the natural social consequences of his own misbehavior, he is in a developmental situation in which aggressiveness usually pays off, and of course this encourages the fixation of an unsocialized aggressive pattern of behavior. With such a fixation the unsocialized aggressive reaction crystallizes into an antisocial personality.

Over the years, I do not believe that the objective in the treatment of the unsocialized aggressive child has changed in any basic way. Additional techniques adaptable to this objective have been developed. Particularly for the younger children behavior modification, skillfully planned, can control abrasive aspects of behavior. Group pressures and group therapy in peer groups may be helpful with those who are not so hostile or rejecting as to invite scapegoating by the group, for the fundamental problem is to extend personal acceptance while pressure is maintained for the modification of behavior. This can really test the breadth and depth of one's humanity.

CHAPTER 8

THE SOCIALIZED DELINQUENT

("We make our own rules!")

EVERY SOCIETY BUILDS ITS RULES OR LAWS, FOR WITHOUT RULES
NO SOCIETY CAN EXIST. THE SIMPLEST ORGANIZATION IS THAT STEM-
MING FROM DOMINANCE OF A SINGLE INDIVIDUAL—THE PATTERN OF
THE DICTATOR. THIS PATTERN NECESSARILY LEAVES MOST, IF NOT
ALL, OTHER INDIVIDUALS INSECURE AND VULNERABLE, AND CONSE-
QUENTLY, IT IS TRADITIONALLY A RELATIVELY UNSTABLE FORM OF
ORGANIZATION, FOR IT FAILS TO GIVE MANY INDIVIDUALS A SECURE
STAKE IN THE SYSTEM AND IN ITS CONTINUANCE.

The evolution of the English language is of real interest
on this point. Webster defines *right* as that side of the body
which is usually the stronger. One's rights, originally, were what
one had the power to take and to hold.

But force alone cannot build a stable society, for as soon as
an "out" becomes strong enough, he will make himself the "in,"
and an unorganized society has no limits on reprisals. A stable
society requires some moral sanctions, some effective respect for
"I ought" as well as "I can." Activating the verb "ought" depends
upon recognizing some mutuality of obligation. For human
relations go more smoothly and more satisfactorily when rights
are not simply enforced by the strong against the weak, but
when a mutuality of obligation is recognized. Unilateral rights
of the strong over the weak tend to be replaced by bilateral
rights, or co-rights which are not unilateral but are symmetrical.
For people need each other, and human cooperation is easier
to maintain when there is some mutual respect, some turn-about.
This principle was embodied in the doctrine of co-rights, which

are to be mutually respected. Behavior which respected co-rights was recognized as *correct* behavior. The individual who could not be prevailed upon or educated to respect co-rights was pronounced *incorrigible* and was killed or banished.

To some degree, it is perhaps inevitable that the rules always tend to favor those with the greater possessions, the greater power. Anatole France wrote: "The Law, with its majestic equality, forbids the rich, as well as the poor, to sleep under bridges, to beg in the streets and to steal." And almost inevitably, the law tends somewhat to favor the generation which has reached the zenith of its power over the young. However, equality before the law is a desirable ideal, and if we do not reach it in practice, at least our effort to do so, destroys the grosser and cruder kinds of exploitation of power.

If our complex civilization is to survive, it is necessary that the young learn from the elders the techniques that make its continuance possible. This requires a discipline of work—a discipline which some are reluctant to learn. The time they are expected to learn it is a time of restlessness, of adventurousness and uncertainty, and a time when their material rewards for effort, although substantial, are usually less than those of the older generation.

The generation gap is not new but, with the wealth of communication presently available by magazine, by television and radio, by phonograph records, and with the massing of the young in schools and on college campuses, it has been accentuated, and we have become more aware of it.

One of the characteristics of man as a social animal is his tendency to ally himself with others in an action group for common purposes. In some remote sense, the modern urban delinquent gang is a descendant of the ancient hunting group's mutual aid and loyalty. A gang evolves as a result of shared experiences. Casual cooperation between delinquent boys in acts of delinquency often leads to increasing definition of a gang, with group members, fringers and those wholly outside the group.

A gang requires of its members a basic capacity for teamwork and for sharing. It requires courage, loyalty, and a measure of dependability.

The socialized delinquents form the best-marked cluster among Ackerson IJR cases.[25] The cluster for boys includes the characteristics of *stealing, truancy from home, truancy from school, police arrest, staying out late at night, associating with bad companions, "running with a gang," smoking, loitering, lying, incorrigibility,* and *leading others into bad conduct.*

With girls, the central entry is *staying out late at night.* The second, third and fourth entries for girls, *truancy from home, truancy from school and police arrest* are identical with those for boys. Then appear *lying, sex delinquency, stealing, over-interest in opposite sex, incorrigibility, associating with bad companions* and *loitering.*

It should be evident, as is well-known, that while delinquent activity with boys focuses most often on stealing, delinquent activity with girls, at least as society presently defines delinquent activity with girls, focuses on night hours and sexual activity.

Hilda Lewis, in her follow-up of children who had been in the Mersham Reception Center[32] found socialized delinquency associated with parental neglect and bad peer-group company.

The computer reworking of some Ann Arbor material[12] defined the socialized delinquent group as those showing at least three of the traits: *furtive stealing, cooperative stealing, running away from home overnight, habitual truancy from school, association with undesirable companions,* and *petty stealing.* There were 53 cases which met these criteria, and did not show more traits of any other cluster. Ninety-one per cent were boys. The interquartile age range was the highest of all the groups: 12 to 15 years.

Staying out late at night and *gang activities* were significantly high in this socialized delinquent group. Background factors were the *low educational level of both parents,* the *working mother, the large family (eight or more children in the home),* the *unkempt dwelling exterior, irregularity of meals, work, retiring,* and *lack of supervision of children's activities.* The absent father, the deceased father, and the *alcoholic father person* were all disproportionately frequent.

The study of Kobayashi *et al.*[30] found the socialized delinquents the best defined cluster of all. The "primary symptoms" were recorded as *association with undesirable companions, cooperative stealing,* and *gang activities.* They recorded the "secondary symptoms" as *stealing from home and/or school, staying out late at night,* and *running away from home overnight.* The "peripheral symptoms" were *occasional truancy from school in the past, habitual truancy from school, assaultive tendencies, deceptiveness, unkindness, general lack of self-control,* and *smoking.*

In the IJR material of 1,500 cases[14, 15] socialized delinquency was determined in terms of the presence of at least two of seven entries. One of these had to be one of the four behavioral entries of *solitary stealing, group stealing, truancy from school, running away from home.* The second entry necessary for inclusion might be another one of these four or might be the psychiatrist's judgment that the primary problem area was *socially unacceptable acts,* his judgment that the relationship made by the child with the psychiatrist was *guarded, defensive, resistive,* or the psychologist's judgment that the relationship made by the child with the psychologist was *guarded, defensive, resistive, suspicious.*

There were 231 socialized delinquents so defined among 1,500 children. This group of 231 delinquents includes 59 (88 per cent) of the 67 children with the entry *running away from home* and 38 (84 per cent) of the 45 with the entry group *stealing.* It includes 92 (79 per cent) of 116 children with the entry *truancy from school* and 157 (73 per cent) of the 215 children with the entry *solitary stealing.* It included 158 (57 per cent) of the 276 cases in which the psychiatrist considered the primary problem area to be *socially unacceptable acts,* 77 (37 per cent) of the 209 cases in which the relationship made by the child with the psychiatrist was rated by the latter as *guarded, defensive, resistive,* and 31 (31 percent) of 101 instances in which the child's relationship to the psychological examiner was rated by the latter as *guarded, defensive, suspicious, resistive.*

The children classified as socialized delinquents tend to be beyond the age of 10 when first seen, and are a much larger portion of those over 14 than of those who are younger. Black children are over-represented in our material.

A disproportionately smaller number of socialized delinquent children have both their natural parents in the home. The parents are likely to be separated or divorced, with the child living with his natural mother and a stepfather.

Selectively these children come from families of four and more children. Middle children are over-represented, the youngest under-represented.

Referral is typically by a court, sometimes a social agency. Medical referrals are unusual.

There is some excess of fathers whose religion is listed as "undetermined."

The principal informant is likely to be someone other than the parents. The mother is likely to be non-accepting of the referral.

The family is likely to be receiving economic assistance or is in need, if not being assisted.

The pregnancy was typically unplanned. The developmental history has more than the usual number of "unknown" entries. Infantile speech is infrequently reported in the developmental history.

The child is less likely than the average clinic child to have a room alone and is more likely to have a bed with a sibling of the same sex.

Compared with the clinic parents in general, these parents stress *withdrawal of privileges* as a means of punishment, with *physical punishment, physical restraint or confinement* and *extra chores* also stressed.

The social history reveals previous parental conflict more frequently than with the average clinic child. The mother is likely not to have been married to the father when the child was conceived.

The mother's attitude toward the child at the time of examination, as judged by the social worker, is likely to be characterized as: *overt rejection; delegates parental responsibility to others; punitive; marked preference for sibling; cold, distant, neglectful* or *acting out through child*. It is unlikely to be characterized as *infantilizing, overprotective*. The father's attitude is characterized as *controlling, rigid* or as *acting out through child*. (The characterizations of the father as *cold, distant, neglectful* and *punitive* are also significantly more frequent than in the general clinic population.)

The social history reveals that the mother is likely to have come from a *broken home*. With a disproportionate frequency the social worker characterizes the mother's area of difficulty as *delinquency or promiscuity*. Paternal *alcoholism* is significantly more frequent than in the clinic population as a whole.

The psychologist is unlikely to find, in his examination, symptomatic evidence of *organic impairment or deficit* or of *speech impairment*. The psychologist sees his relationship with the environment as *acting out*, not as *withdrawn, passive*. Manifestation of hostility is *excessive—easily elicited*. The child's relationship with his parents is described as *hostile-aggressive*, not as *submissive*.

Aside from the elements of behavior on which these cases were elected, the psychiatrist lists as problems *lying, disobedience with hostile component, firesetting* and *destructiveness*. Under personality difficulties he lists *bullying, domineering, aggressive* and selectively avoids *withdrawn, seclusive, daydreaming* and *overly conforming, submissive*.

Dynamic factors, as judged by the psychiatrist, include *more than one placement in the past*.

In the psychiatrist's judgment the mother's reaction to the child's primary problem is very unlikely to be *overanxious* and very likely to be *indifferent, detached, minimized*. The mother's relationship with the child is characterized as *cold, distant, neglectful*, as *overt rejection*, as *acting out through child*, or as *punitive* in that order. It is not *infantilizing, overprotective*. The paternal relationship with the child is characterized as *acting out through the child*. It is not likely to be either *reasonably wholesome* nor *overly seductive*, nor is the paternal reaction to the child's primary problem likely to be *reasonably concerned*. The nature of the relationship is further indicated by the fact that *overt rejection* by the father and the *delegation of parental responsibility to others* reach significance. Paternal *irresponsibility, poor work record* is used to characterize the father. Paternal *alcoholism, delinquency* and *minimal information or unknown* are also significantly frequent in this group.

Neither parent is accepting of the concept of self-involvement in the patient's problem. The attitude of the mother concerning therapy for herself is *reluctant, resistant, refusing.* The parental relationship is not likely to be *reasonably satisfactory* and is likely to show *marked overt parental conflict.*

In the intake study at Iowa City[28] we compared 25 children classified as socialized delinquents with the remaining 275 cases.

The socialized delinquents typically were referred at older ages than the other children. They were referred by the juvenile court after trouble with the law or occasionally by a social agency after an instance of destructiveness or overaggressive behavior.

The parents did not consistently check any descriptive terms for their children but did selectively *omit* checking *affectionate* and *sensitive.* It seems logical to assume that they tended to see these children as unaffectionate and insensitive. A number had run away from home. Truancy from school was typical.

The mothers of these children were typically young mothers in good health during pregnancy. Toilet training and speech development typically presented no special problems. These families often had lost the father through death.

Both parents typically reported that no member of the family was very close to any other member. The child's relation to his siblings was generally indifferent to poor. The father reported that the father-child relationship involved more conflict than harmony. The parents reported that when "in a jam" the child turned "to no one" and specifically that he did *not* turn to either parent.

In a further study of the 1,500 IJR cases,[14, 15] a comparison was made of socialized delinquents with the unsocialized aggressive children. It was at once evident that the unsocialized aggressive children were typically referred at younger ages, were more frequently white, were more frequently medical referrals, and less frequently court referrals. All of these differences washed out when we compared a smaller group of cases matched on age and sex. Items which persisted in the matched groups indicated that the socialized delinquents came from larger and poorer families than the unsocialized aggressive children. They were less likely to have a room alone, more likely to have been exposed to sex activity, and less likely to have been bladder trained by the second birthday.

Ignoring the items on which the groups were selected, the unsocialized aggressive children were much more likely to be disobedient, even omitting the instances classified as *disobedience with hostile component,* much more likely than the socialized delinquent to be classified by the psychiatrist as showing *personality difficulties* as the primary problem area. The chief problem was classified as "frequent or constant," rather than "occasional," as was the case with the socialized delinquent; and the psychiatrist was notably more likely to regard the unsocialized aggressive children as *severely disturbed.* The psychiatrist was notably more inclined to consider the unsocialized aggressive children as *restless, excitable,* while the social history was more likely to describe the socialized delinquent as having had no difficulties with speech, and the psychologist was more likely to report no unusual patterning in the psychological tests. The unsocialized aggressive child was more likely to be described as *generally immature,* despite this matching for age and sex, and *overly competitive* with other children.

Even with the small number of cases which could be matched for age and sex, certain maternal problems are recorded reliably more frequently with the mothers of the unsocialized aggressive children. These include the mother whose reaction to the child's problem is *overanxious,* the mother whose relation with the child is *controlling, rigid,* and the mother who shows a *marked preference for a sibling.*

If we contrast the unsocialized aggressive children in the intake information study with the socialized delinquents in that study,[29] several significant relations appear.

The parents are prone to describe the unsocialized aggressive child as *cruel.*

While the socialized delinquent is accepted as an equal by his peer group, the unsocialized aggressive child is likely *not* to be so accepted.

The socialized delinquent is unlikely to turn to his father when in a jam. The unsocialized aggressive child is significantly more likely to do so.

It seems clear that the socialized delinquent is typically a product of the large, impoverished family unable to offset the influence of a delinquency area on an otherwise normal child, while the unsocialized aggressive child appears to a greater extent to be the product of a family pathology, and, specifically, of an unsatisfactory mother-child relationship.

The typical problem with the socialized delinquent lies not in any maternal or parental lack of basic affectional acceptance of the child. Rather it lies in the lack of effective supervision and control of the older child, and frequently also—for the boys especially—in a lack of an adequate adult masculine pattern to emulate. Growing up in an overcrowded home in a delinquent area without sufficient adult attention or control, these children fall into a street gang, which becomes a delinquent gang by a natural process of growth. This is an example more of neighborhood pathology than of individual psychopathology.

Of course, establishing the existence of a cluster of correlated symptoms such as constitute the syndrome of socialized delinquency does not mean that this cluster cannot be subdivided. A complete clustering of data from 300 delinquent youths in the New York State Training School for Boys (Warwick) yielded three clusters.[22] The unsocialized aggressive cluster came through in usual style, but it was found possible to subdivide the socialized delinquent into a larger truly socialized group focusing on group delinquent activity, and a smaller poorly socialized group focusing on repeated running away from home overnight. These runaway children prove to be the fringers of the delinquent group. This division made us examine further those cases known to have been involved in *group stealing* and those cases known to be involved in *running away from home overnight*. The next two chapters will deal with these sub-groups.

CHAPTER 9

THE GROUP DELINQUENT REACTION
(The Predatory Gang)

Our computer study of the Warwick boys[22] mentioned earlier made it clear that the socialized delinquent cluster as we had described it, was divisible into two clusters, one relating to the "group delinquent" reaction and the other to the "runaway" reaction.

One cluster showed 89 boys out of the 300 with four or more of the following intercorrelated traits:

	Incidence in 300 cases
Stealing	92%
Undesirable companions	74%
Cooperative stealing	59%
Gang activity	40%
Gambling	12%

As nearly all boys in the training school had been involved in stealing, this trait had little differential usefulness. However, all of the other entries involved relations with others and, typically, involvement with them in delinquent activities. These boys were usually with both parents (91 per cent) and were more inclined toward aggressive stealing than the other groups. Here is one instance:

Ned was committed to the state training school for delinquent boys at the age of 15.

Ned was the youngest of four boys. Both his parents were high school dropouts who married at the beginning of the American involvement in World War II. It was Ned's father's second marriage. Subsequently this man served 4 years in the U.S. Army and was decorated for bravery. However, he had a serious drinking problem and deserted his family after 14 years. Two years later Ned's mother remarried. She had one child by her second husband, a boy who died of pneumonia at age 3. This marriage was terminated by divorce after six years.

The position of a woman alone trying to raise teen-age sons is a difficult one at best, and Ned's mother was not able to control her boys. She herself had a drinking problem and was a very permissive, overprotective mother. It was reported that at an early age her boys were exposed to open sex relations in the home when she would come home intoxicated with men friends. At the age of 10 Ned was found stealing from a store a quantity of caps for his cap pistol. He was warned by the police. He was subsequently known to steal a lady's purse from a coat rack. At the age of 14 he was arrested with several other boys for stealing money from a service station. However, there was not enough evidence to file charges, and some of the money was recovered. Two months later, he was first in Juvenile Court after he broke into a cafe with three companions and stole a 32 caliber pistol from the cash drawer. It was learned that he had also been involved in stealing money from the public library. He was put on probation. The boy and his mother were referred to a mental health center which made some efforts toward treatment for five months, apparently without much success and closed the case.

Two months after his court appearance, Ned knocked a 7th grade boy unconscious. Ned maintained that this boy had been picking on a slightly retarded boy and the matter was dropped with Ned's paying $55 dollars' expenses for x-rays, etc. from the funds he was earning in the youth program. Apparently, in terms of adolescent boy standards, the assault was not wholly unprovoked.

Eight months later at age 15 Ned, with another boy, broke into a private home and stole whiskey. Ned lied about this in court, but his companion confessed and later Ned admitted his own involvement. Probation was continued. Ten months later at age 16, Ned was caught in the public library trying to break into the safe after having broken into the building. Placement in a group home was considered in the Juvenile Court. The next day Ned was found selling stolen tickets for a high school play and was committed to the state training school for delinquent boys.

Ned and his three brothers were all school dropouts. At the time Ned was committed to the training school, his oldest brother, age 20, was under a suspended sentence for forgery and was a known heroin addict. His next brother, at 18, had been twice in the state training school for delinquent boys and was currently in the young men's reformatory for an armed robbery committed while on parole from the training school. Ned's next older brother, age 17, had been in the state juvenile home for dependent and neglected children twice and had run away numerous times.

It was clear from conversations with Ned that, as is usually the case with the more experienced delinquent, his court record, like the surface of the iceberg, is only the part that shows. Ned was actively involved with four or five others in burglarizing a number of places. Except for the assault, his delinquencies were all committed with others.

Ned's verbal IQ was bright normal, while his performance IQ was in the superior range. The psychologist noted, among other things:

> He is a witty lad and has learned to use his quick ability to amuse others to buy time—for himself. It is hard not to fall into the trap, for his spontaneous witticisms are so quick and so pertinent, as well as in good taste, that one responds to that rather than to the fact that it is a delaying and bribery tactic. It has evidently been a most successful tool for Ned, for he uses it consistently within the described context. Ned's very good vocabulary serves him well in this as well as in other situations.

Ned's performance on a Miale-Holsopple sentence completion test, given blind to a skilled interpreter of sentence completions among a number of completions by patients on an adolescent ward in a state hospital, proved interesting. The blind interpretation was as follows: socialized, intelligent, not hostile, not aggressive, reserved, interested in the world, observes clearly and accurately. Why is this patient hospitalized?

Clearly Ned has a number of assets, including good intelligence and real social skills. His more or less dependable loyalties are probably limited to his mother and to his delinquent associates. It is clear that he has little guilt over his delinquencies. The chances are that he will come to realize that crime does not often pay as well—in the long run—as steady employment. When he comes to this realization, he will probably give up his delinquent behavior, if not suddenly, then at least gradually. Hopefully this may occur before he has a criminal conviction in the adult court.*

In our 1,500 IJR cases[14, 15] the entry *group stealing* was included. We had only 45 children *known* to have been involved in group stealing among our 1,500 IJR cases. This number is small, and if our information were more complete, our results would doubtless be better. However, since group stealing is typically a central element in the group delinquent reaction, it seems desirable to study the comparisons.

It was notable but certainly not surprising that group stealing occurred particularly in those over 14 years of age. Ninth graders were over-represented. Although these children tended to be a shade older than the runaways, more of them were slow in their grade progress in school. Five out of the six were boys, as compared with three boys to one girl in the clinic population as a whole. Families of less than three children were at a deficit in this group, while families of more than three children were disproportionately frequent. The middle children were particularly likely to be involved, probably by reason of the fact that their position is more apt to result in reduced parental attention. Eight of the 45 children had run away from home, which indicates the tendency of these problems to flow together. However, in contrast with the runaway children, these children showed no special problems of firesetting or promiscuity. *Fear*

---

* Ned was paroled after not quite seven months in the training school. After four months in the community he seemed to be doing quite well. He was doing well in high school. His relationship with his mother was distinctly improved, and probably was aided by some sessions of family therapy conducted by his counselor at the Training School who continued his contacts with Ned and his mother after Ned returned home. One of Ned's brothers at this time was in college, one in Bible school, and one in the state reformatory.

of school or reluctance to attend was not more frequent than the clinic average.

Compared with the clinic average, these children were infrequently described as *withdrawn, seclusive, daydreaming,* as *generally immature* or as *chronically anxious or fearful.*

As with the runaways and unsocialized aggressives, court referrals were frequent, medical referrals infrequent.

Also as with the runaways the relationship of the child with the psychological examiner tended to be *guarded, defensive, resistive, suspicious.*

The economic situation of the home was frequently worse even than is the case with the runaway child in that there was likely to be need and *no* assistance. *Marked economic problems* in the home were frequent.

In contrast to the family of the runaway, which was often broken by separation or divorce, these families had a disproportionate number of parents lost by death.

Housing was crowded and these children were exposed to sex activity significantly more frequently than the clinic average.

The mothers were unlikely to be overanxious about the child's problem but were inclined to be protective or defensive. They were likely to be non-accepting of the referral or at least ambivalent toward it.

The family discipline was not unusual except for a greater-than-usual frequency of prolonged punishment.

In the judgment of the social worker, the fathers were often *critical, depreciative,* often *punitive,* and often *pushing the child to early responsibility.* The mother was inclined to be *overly permissive* and to *delegate parental responsibility to others.* The father was inclined to *alcoholism, delinquency* more frequently than the clinic average.

By contrast with the families of the runaways, the cold, distant neglectful mother and the overtly rejecting mother were uncommon here. A tyrannical marital partner, usually the father, was not uncommon.

Studies at the Iowa Training School for Boys[43, 45] revealed a notably more normal profile on the Minnesota Multiphasic

Personality Inventory for these cooperative delinquents than for either the runaway or the unsocialized aggressive groups. These boys have notably better child-parent and parent-child relations as revealed in the Parent-Child Relations Questionnaire and notably a much more favorable self-image than the unsocialized aggressive, and doubtless than the runaway delinquents as well.

The current conflict with their parents is typically the result of adolescent rebellion and the delinquency itself. The parents can usually be worked with successfully, and family therapy sessions are often quite successful.

These boys are not difficult to like and they are often quite responsive to an interested, understanding man.

The treatment of the socialized delinquent was discussed in Chapter 8.

It is noteworthy that *Brothers in Crime*[41] by Clifford Shaw is an excellent case study.

CHAPTER 10

THE RUNAWAY REACTION

("Run-run-run")

RUNNING AWAY IS AN UNDERSTANDABLE WAY OF DEALING WITH A SITUATION ONE CANNOT MASTER OR MANAGE AND, IN SOME INSTANCES, IS EVEN A VERY APPROPRIATE COURSE. THE RUNAWAY REACTION RELATES TO REPETITIVE RUNNING AWAY FROM HOME OVERNIGHT OR LONGER. IT USUALLY INDICATES THAT THE CHILD IS EXTREMELY UNHAPPY IN HIS HOME, AND THAT FOR HIM HOME IS MORE OF A THREAT THAN A REFUGE. THIS, IN TURN, IS AN INDICATION THAT HE FEELS THE PEOPLE IN THE HOME ARE CRITICAL OR THREATENING, RATHER THAN SUPPORTING.

Reference has been made to our computer study of Warwick boys (cf. Chapter 9) and the cluster of traits characterizing the group delinquent reaction. A second cluster, characterizing the unsocialized aggressive reaction, was also evident. The third cluster centered around the following entries:

	Incidence in 300 cases
Staying out late at night	54%
Repeatedly running away from home overnight	53%
Furtive stealing	51%
Stealing in the home	29%
Passive homosexuality	10%

These are delinquent acts of a timid, furtive, or fugacious type. In fact there were 61 cases with at least three such entries.*

---

* In order to keep up with the size of our group, we required only three entries instead of the four that were required for the group delinquents. Had we required four, the number would have been substantially smaller.

We have already considered the cluster of unsocialized aggressive delinquency in Chapter 7.

Computer clustering is perhaps most useful when it clarifies and forces us to take account of what we already know but have failed to see in perspective. The tough, aggressive hostile delinquent stands out and forces himself on our recognition. He stands alone. The competent member of the juvenile gang forces himself on our attention in his own right. But the timid, furtive chronic runaway boy does not stand alone and tends to disappear into the outer fringes of the delinquent gang, where he is tolerated and used when such use is convenient. He is not really accepted as a member of the gang, as he is undependable. In his inner hostility and resentment, he resembles the unsocialized aggressive boy, although he lacks his toughness and his courage. He is not truly a socialized delinquent, but because he is a misfit he becomes a hanger-on to a delinquent group and clusters with this group in some of his behavior traits. The unsocialized aggressive and the chronic runaway are *both* basically unsocialized and their behavior resembles the alternatives of fight or flight emphasized by Walter Cannon.

The following case is illustrative, although most cases of the runaway reaction respond more favorably to treatment than this one did.

Dan was the youngest of seven children born to an unstable woman who was apparently slightly retarded mentally.

When Dan was two years old, he lost his father. Dan's mother remarried, divorced, and remarried again. Her third husband was sentenced to prison for sexual involvement with Dan's sister. When Dan was eight, his mother died and Dan and his sister were placed with a brother of Dan's mother. This uncle was married and the couple had two daughters, one and two years older than Dan. This uncle was later reported to have punished Dan severely on occasions, beating him with belt buckles which left bruises. He drank to excess and was not a good provider. The aunt was a poor housekeeper. Dan's sister soon married and left the home. Dan's uncle and his wife separated periodically.

When Dan was 9½ his sister reported to the ADC worker that

she felt Dan should be removed from the aunt's home because he was being mistreated. She said Dan was knocked down the stairs by his aunt and that she had beaten him several times. Apparently nothing was done at this time and a month later the aunt reported to the Police Department that Dan had run away. He was found three days later by a neighbor, riding a stolen bicycle. When his aunt left the home to call the police and report that Dan had been found, he ran away again and was picked up by the police two days later and taken to the Juvenile Home.

Dan said that he ran away from home because he constantly feared severe punishment. Apparently there was factual basis for his fear although he was known to lie a great deal, some of his lies bordering on fantasy.

Dan was seen at the Juvenile Home by a psychologist from the Guidance Center. He was regarded as a very deprived youngster who was immature and easily became silly in his behavior, but was also bitter and vindictive toward his aunt, feeling that she rejected him.

At ten years of age Dan was placed by the Juvenile Court in the care and custody of a good child-placing agency. He then was placed in a foster home and remained there approximately three and one-half months. His behavior was reported to be quite babyish and demanding and resistant to discipline. He seemed to expect to be treated like his two foster brothers, ages 3 and 4. He started scaring them and abusing them sexually. He was removed on the request of the foster parents and placed in a group home. He was then just 11. Less than three weeks later he ran away from the group home with another boy and they later stole a car. The boys were apprehended and Dan was returned to the group home. He attended public school. He was involved in stealing four bicycles. Three were recovered and he was making payments on the fourth from his allowance. The school principal and other school officials interested in Dan bought him a bicycle. For a time he seemed to be responding well to his caseworker. However, he began to have uncontrollable temper outbursts and to fight excessively with other children, demanding to be removed from the group home, and threatening to set fire to the home. He did set fire to a pile of his clothing in his room. This fire caused considerable damage.

Dan was committed to the children's unit at a state mental hospital. Here he was found at 12 years of age to test at the low average level in intelligence. His responses on projective tests were those of a self-centered and anxious youngster who felt weak, inferior, and inadequate. He gave evidence of affectional deprivation and feelings of rejection. There was marked hostility and there were aggressive fantasies. He had a low tolerance for frustration and tended to act impulsively. He lacked a sense of personal responsibilty and appeared to feel that he should be cared for by someone else.

He was enrolled in an active program of individual psychotherapy but seemed not really able to establish a meaningful relation with his therapist or to trust the therapist enough to confide in him. He presented some problems of adjustment on the ward, with peers, in school and in recreation periods. In a review after he had been 4 months in the hospital it was noted: "The most significant problems in the total hospital program have been the boy's marked immaturity, impulsivity and his inability to involve himself with meaningful adults. Apparently this boy has a long history of severe rejection and at this time does not have the ability to trust adults to a degree that will allow him to become closely involved with them."

Another review 8 months later was more favorable. He was able to relate better to his therapist and his agency worker and to maintain minimal but sustained improvement. His peer relationships remained poor, however. He was discharged after a year of hospitalization to a foster home placement which pleased him. It was felt that he had made only minimum progress, but that he had obtained maximum hospital benefit.

Despite some initial testing behavior, Dan did quite well in the foster home for a time. He became quite insecure over the prospect of a natural son in the family returning from service in Viet Nam. This crisis passed successfully, but then his foster parents took a handicapped baby into their home. Dan could not tolerate competing for attention with a younger child. During his second year in the foster home his behavior began to deteriorate. He would steal at home. At the school bus stop he was reported to bother other children to a point where mothers in the neighborhood were walking their children to the bus. He was reported to show off by recklessly jumping in front of cars on the highway. In task assignments he was undependable, a show-off and constantly interrupted the conversation of others.

After 17 months he was returned to the children's unit of the mental hospital because of the deterioration in his behavior. Again he had individual psychotherapy, a remedial school program, and a closely structured work and recreation program. Again there was slow improvement, although he continued to act as a boy three or four years younger. He still had particular difficulty with peer relations and would do best in a one-to-one relation with a staff member. His foster parents visited him monthly and his social worker visited him every two weeks.

After seven months in the children's unit he was returned to his foster home. He made an adjustment in school, but complained that his foster parents were somewhat critical of him, and that this made him uncomfortable. After four months he was found by his foster parents trying to take the panties off a seven year old neighbor girl. With this, the foster parents gave up and Dan was returned to the Juvenile Home. A month later he was placed in a farm foster home. Here he adjusted fairly well initially, except for a transient problem of school truancy. He took some interest in farm work, but still tended to let things slide and then hide the fact from the foster parents. After 11 months he was returned to the group home. After two weeks he ran away. He was picked up two days later and placed in the Juvenile Home. After ten days he was returned to the group home. Eight days later he ran away again. He was picked up in a neighboring state three days later. A petition of delinquency was filed at this time.

While in the Juvenile Home he broke a window and incited a disturbance which resulted in seven boys, including Dan, being transferred to jail. After three days he was returned to the Juvenile Home on his promise of good behavior. Dan had a hearing with an attorney representing him and he was released to live at the YMCA. He stayed only one night at the Y and did not report for the job which had been arranged. He then began to bother his former foster mother and her neighbors with requests for money, cigarettes, the use of the car, etc. He was arrested in a stolen car, which was found to be the 12th he had taken. He was committed to the Iowa Training School for Boys.

Dan's verbal IQ was 99, his performance IQ, 100, and his full scale IQ on the Wexler Adult Intelligence Scale, 100. He showed some evidence of rigidity in his thinking. He had been attending the 9th grade, but his actual achievement ranged from 3.8 in language to 7.2 in arithmetic applications.

Dan was in the Training School for 10 months on this commitment. He did not adjust well. He alienated other boys by lying and stealing from them. He worked in the kitchen and made some progress, but his personal relationships were shallow. He had a trial visit out of the Training School at Christmas and visited with the family of his kitchen work supervisor, but ran away. He was picked up by the local police and returned to the Training School and spent 18 days in the detention unit.

After ten months in the Training School Dan was paroled to live in a group home and work in a tree nursery. During his first month he took off in a nursery truck, drove to his home city, a distance of about 30 miles, visited a store where his aunt had formerly shopped, located her sister through the store, and through this sister located his aunt. He phoned his aunt, picked her up at work, drove her home and had supper with her. He told his aunt that he was living at the group home and working at the nursery and that he had the truck for the weekend. Following this incident Dan was returned to the Training School. He was permitted to work at seasonal work with a local company. He stole a truck and took off, but put that truck in a ditch. He was picked up by training school staff and spent three weeks in the detention unit before being returned to his cottage. Less than a month later when permitted to attend a Bible camp, he took off in a panel truck. Two days later he was picked up in a nearby city and returned to the detention unit. Until about a year ago, he was still in the training school.

Obviously this boy's future remains problematical. He has been profoundly egocentric, and he remains so. His focus is so much on a deprived "poor me" that he does not clearly perceive his own contribution to his continuing problem. He cannot get

outside the prison of his egocentricity and his impulsive irrespon-
sible behavior continues. When he sees a motor vehicle that he
can drive, he takes it. However, when other treatment efforts
fail, Father Time tends to make a gradual contribution. Even
the unstable become less reckless as they grow older. We can
hope, as well as continue our efforts.*

A computer analysis[22] of material from the case records of
300 delinquents in the New York State Training School for Boys
revealed a cluster of traits including *staying out late at night,
repeatedly running away from home overnight, furtive stealing,
stealing in the home,* and *passive homosexuality.* Sixty-one boys,
among the 300 having at least three of these entries, were
included in a runaway cluster.

Notably, the group delinquents generally do their stealing
away from home, while the runaway child is particularly prone
to steal in the home, sometimes as a preparation for running
away, as when he steals his father's pay and takes off. The
runaway children are likely to engage solely in furtive stealing,
sneak-thief activity, while the group delinquents, as well as the
unsocialized aggressive, are more prone to turn to aggressive
stealing such as burglary. The runaway boys are more likely
than other delinquents to be at the receiving end of homosexual
activity, sometimes to gain favors or protection.

The analysis revealed that the degree of family pathology
is maximal in the runaway boys, somewhat less with the unsocialized aggressive, and least with the cooperative delinquents
who come within the definition of the *group delinquent reaction.*
Six indices of family pathology included the status of the *unwanted child, parental rejection, illegitimacy, only child status,
child presently in other family,* and present or past *foster family
placement.* In all of these the average status of the group
delinquents was the most favorable, the runaway child the least
favorable.

---

* Twenty-one months after his admission Dan was given a direct discharge.
He was at that time eighteen years of age, and it was believed that further efforts
in the Training School to treat him as a juvenile delinquent would not be helpful.
Five months later an inquiry received from the Men's Reformatory indicated
that he had been committed there for stealing a motor vehicle.

The boys in the runaway cluster were particularly prone to *emotional immaturity, apathy* and *seclusiveness.* It is clear that the runaway delinquents usually have a very bad self-image. The runaway reaction represents a frustration response of maladaptive delinquency, while the group delinquent reaction is a more adaptive type of delinquency implying less personal and family pathology. Two studies[43, 45] at the Iowa Training School for Boys reveal more pathology in the Minnesota Multiphasic Personality Inventory for the runaway boys and for the unsocialized aggressive boys than for the group delinquents. The Parent-Child Relations Questionnaire, or PCR, clearly indicates poorer child-parent and parent-child relations for the runaway and unsocialized aggressive boys than for the group delinquents.

If, in the IJR material,[14, 15] we compare 67 children recorded to have run away from home overnight with 1,433 cases with no such entry, a number of interesting relationships become evident.

It is obvious that runaway children are rebellious, and it is certainly not surprising that they frequently become involved in delinquencies other than running away. They face the problem of maintaining themselves on runaway, and inevitably they fall into association with other delinquent children and learn from them. They are frequently involved in *truancy from school,* in *solitary stealing,* occasionally in *group stealing,* and their rebelliousness toward authority is frequently expressed in *disobedience with a hostile component.* Not infrequently these runaway children have preferred to associate with older children. Nine were known to have been involved in *firesetting,* and six were described as *promiscuous.* In these last two entries they contrasted strongly with the clinic population as a whole, and somewhat with the 45 children involved in group stealing, as the latter had only two individuals who had been involved in firesetting and only two who were described as promiscuous.

The sex ratio of the runaways was not different from the clinic average, which would indicate that, while boys are more prone than girls to the *group delinquent reaction* and the *unsocialized aggressive reaction,* yet those girls who come to the clinic are neither more nor less prone to the *runaway reaction* than boys. Black children are over-represented in the *runaway reaction.*

These children usually did not like school, and among them there was a significantly higher than usual incidence of *fear of school,* or *reluctance to attend.*

These children have little occasion to trust adults, and *lying* is characteristic. The psychologist was likely to report the child to be *guarded, defensive, resistive, suspicious.* Typically, the child manifested *excessive hostility, easily elicited.* The psychologist with a disproportionately high frequency judged these children to be *severely disturbed.*

Naturally, the proportion of runaways who were referred by courts was high and the proportion of medical referrals was low.

Young children do not often run away from home overnight. In the runaway group there was an excess of children over 14 years of age and in the tenth to twelfth grades. Compared with the clinic average, this group contained an excess of black children, a finding which doubtless related to the high incidence of family disorganization in the black community.

The runaway is especially prone to occur in the home broken by separation or divorce and when the mother is the only parental figure. Selectively families receiving public assistance were over-represented in the runaway group.

Compared with the clinic average, there was a greater than usual frequency of mothers not married to the father at the time this child was conceived. The unplanned pregnancy was over-represented, the planned pregnancy relatively infrequent.

The degree of maternal maturity and the family situation were not supporting of maternal behavior, and the mother who was described as *cold, distant, neglectful* and the mother who was described as *overtly rejecting* were decidedly over-represented in this group. These mothers were *not* overanxious about the child's problem. Although they were likely to talk over much about the child's problem, they tended not to accept their own involvement in it and generally they were not accessible to treatment.

Lack of money was a reason given for the marital maladjustment common in the parental marriage. Not infrequently the mother herself had a problem of delinquency or promiscuity, the father either this or alcoholism. A stepfather was more than usually frequent in the family.

Often these children had been exposed to sexual activity in the home.

A lack of parental wisdom was reflected in the fact that discipline was more than usually likely to include *physical restraint or confinement* and *bribery.* The former suggest unwise severity, and the latter is an invitation to the child to use misbehavior as a source of blackmail.

Herbert Quay, as a result of extensive studies of delinquents, has grouped them in four behavioral categories.[35, 36] His behavioral category 1, the *inadequate-immature* group, has a personality description which resembles that of the *runaway reaction,* even though many of his inadequate-immature delinquents have not—yet—had the courage to run away from home. If the home conditions are not improved, it is safe to predict that many will do so.

The problems of treating the runaway reaction are extremely close to the problem of treating the unsocialized aggressive reaction except for the lesser degree of aggressiveness and the greater fear and dependency. However, when they are with younger or more helpless children, the runaway children may be hostile and very aggressive. Their appetite for attention may seem insatiable, but learning to respect the rights of others proceeds at a snail's pace at best. One must first try to make the child feel reasonably secure in a relationship, and then apply gentle consistent pressure toward a decent respect for the rights of others.

CHAPTER 11

THE WITHDRAWING REACTION

("Leave me alone!")

W HILE THE HUMAN ANIMAL IS A SOCIAL ANIMAL, SOCIAL RESPONSE, TO BE SUSTAINED, NEEDS THE REINFORCEMENT OF SOME SOCIAL REWARDS. IF RELATIONSHIPS WITH OTHERS ARE TOO UNREWARDING AND TOO FRUSTRATING OVER A PERIOD OF TIME, THE INDIVIDUAL MAY WITHDRAW INTO SOLITUDE AND ISOLATION. THE EASE WITH WHICH WITHDRAWAL SETS IN MAY BE IN PART AN INDICATION OF BOTH THE SOCIABILITY AND THE VITAL DRIVE OF THE PERSON. WITHDRAWAL MAY BE EASILY PROVOKED IN THOSE WITH LITTLE SOCIABILITY AND LOW VITAL DRIVE. IT MAY BE EXCEEDINGLY DIFFICULT TO BRING ABOUT IN THE PERSON WITH A HIGH SOCIABILITY AND A STRONG VITAL DRIVE.

Some years ago I wrote on this topic[7] in part as follows:

Traditional religion and biological science seem to agree that man's present perplexity relates to his having achieved a power of choice and discrimination with respect to a wide range of possible courses of action. He evaluates these courses with varying degrees of certainty or perplexity, as good or evil, wise or foolish. While lower forms of life react in simpler and more predictable ways, and with relatively little that we can identify as indecision, man has expanded the size of his skull, the complexity of his brain, and the extent of his understanding. The increasing sweep of his knowledge has given him an extensive mastery of his outer world but faces him with vast new opportunities for confusion in the complicated decisions he must make, and the enormous and increasing complexity of his inner world.

Dr. John Whitehorn has stated that as the stomach is the

organ of indigestion, so the brain is the organ of maladjustment. The improvement shown by many severely disordered schizophrenics following the massive destruction of the operation of prefrontal lobotomy underlines this observation.

Social relationships have increased in complexity and probably the most widespread and urgent problem met by the growing child, is the problem of reconciling the inner demands of individuality on the one hand with the need for the approval and acceptance of others. Social living forces upon us role-playing, and prescribed forms of behavior which make us all, to some degree, "actors" in our daily actions. Social living demands a certain amount of concealment of the self as well as a certain revealing of the self. Some concealment has social sanction in terms of *the Right of Privacy* or the attitude that *It's None of Your Damn Business.* Or at least such a right *used to be* recognized.

Each of us wants to do as he pleases, and each of us wants the approval of others. We resolve this paradox by building into our personalities, desires and ways of behaving which are acceptable to others. To some degree, we really become socialized. If, particularly in early life, our relations with others are warm and satisfying, if our own emotional needs are met by our parents, then it is easy for us to want happiness for others, and the process of socialization proceeds rather easily. We achieve this because we find satisfactions in our contacts with others, which make it not too difficult to mold ourselves according to some more-or-less acceptable social pattern. With varying degrees of success, we delete or repress desires which we learn are unacceptable. And most of us succeed in attaining a more-or-less comfortable existence, an imperfect but workable integration of inner impulses with the expectations of society, an integration adequate to the extent that we are not usually in any intense conflict over opposing tendencies within ourselves.

We remain actors however. We play roles. We conceal what society demands that we conceal, and what we think it wise to conceal, and we reveal ourselves selectively. The balance between what is concealed and what is revealed is socially important. When the ratio of concealment to revealment is too low, the individual is Common, Crude and Uncultured unless he succeeds in making the grade as an ascetic Saint or Mahatma. Such achievement requires so living that he has nothing more than a few body functions which can be considered deserving of concealment, and he must also exercise effective moral and spiritual leadership, to avoid being classified as just plain Uninteresting or a Bore. When the ratio of concealment to revealment is conspicuously and protectively high, we say that the individual has a Poker Face or a Dead Pan, plays them Close to the Chest, and we call him Close-mouthed or Defensive or Suspicious or perhaps just plain Worried. If he overdoes the role-taking to conceal his true self, we call him a Poseur or a Hypocrite. He lives constantly under a sword of Damocles, i.e. The Danger of Being Found Out. Even if he feels justified in his concealment he lives to some extent in the shadow of fear, as does a scout in hostile territory. This may be well tolerated if the danger is slight, or even if the danger is great, when the cause is conceived to be noble. To the extent he feels unjustified in his concealment or in *what* he is concealing, he lives in anxiety as well as in the shadow of fear. For those who are not Saints, or Mahatmas, who are not Crude and Uncultured, and who would prefer not to be just Uninteresting, a constant problem of living is how much to conceal and even how much to venture which is worthy of concealment. Too much venture creates anxiety. Too little contributes to the risk of ennui and boredom.

Short, perhaps, of being Crude and Uncultured there are those personalities which are open and perhaps naive, but with easy outward expression. And short of the Suspicious, the Poseurs or the Hypocrites, there are those who are anxiously and self-consciously guarded and uneasy in their relations with others. And among them we see a disproportionate amount of mental illness develop.

For most of us, the positive social rewards of warmth and sharing outweigh the negative aspects of social exchange—the criticism, the disparagement, the derision. My awareness of differing attitudes toward verbal exchange was stimulated by the remark of an inmate of a prison concerning a certain supervisor. "He's a good man to work with. Why you can work with him all day and he'll never say a word to you." In certain situations verbal exchange is usually hostile or limiting. There are those who expect verbal exchange to be hostile not because of the situation, but because of their own make-up. There are those whose life is dominated by the fear of derision which Abraham Myerson called the derision complex. And there are those who have never experienced warmth and sharing to a degree which makes social exchange worth the risk it carries. Such persons have not found the compensations of the active and inner experience of real social acceptance and interpersonal sharing to make up for the denial of primitive individuality which adjustment to society demands. It is not typically that such persons have been mistreated. It is rather that they have not had a degree of the happy experience of becoming one with a group or partner, of real human sharings, which makes holding a place in a world of people an important objective. Sometimes such a person has been to his parents primarily a possession or a responsibility, rather than a personality who should grow to independent maturity under their care.

Healthy adaptation is the maintenance of a balance and continuity in the personality by adjustment to others and the outside environment. In addition to this kind of adaptation we can recognize another, which is preserving the continuity of the inner mental state by *a protective detachment from the outer world,* of not permitting the stimuli of this world to intrude. This kind of adaptation is widely used as a religious practice in prayer or in contemplation particularly in India. In a minor way we all use it in concentrating our attention for the solution of a problem which reqiures all our resources.

We see the same kind of detachment in a morbid form in schizophrenia. Schizophrenic withdrawal is a detachment of interest and attention from the outer world, particularly from the social world. The patient who shows schizophrenic detachment may respond to words, but he does so at either the primitive level of their literal meaning or in terms of their private meaning for him. He has no human interest in the speaker, and exerts no effort to read or understand him as a person. Human interplay is lost or actively avoided. A part of this may be because human relations have commonly been so disturbing to the inner equilibrium of the patient they are consistently avoided. This is what we see in the autistic child who withdraws from human contact. And a part may be because the patient is preoccupied in struggling with a problem which he cannot solve. This is the case with schizophrenic preoccupation. Yet the former is probably also a factor in schizophrenia.

A study by Joseph Mark of our hospital in the Bronx involved submitting 139 statements to 100 mothers of male schizophrenics and 100 mothers of male non-schizophrenics. In fifteen instances the mothers of schizophrenics agreed with the statement more frequently than the mothers of non-schizophrenics with the difference at the .001 level of probability. I would ask that you listen to these statements as I read them and try to form in your mind's eye a picture of the kind of maternal attitude which would lie behind them:

Children should be taken to and from school until the age of eight just to make sure there are no accidents.

A mother should make it her business to know everything her children are thinking.

If children are quiet for a little while, mother should immediately find out what they are thinking about.

Children should not annoy parents with their unimportant problems.

A devoted mother has no time for social life.

A watchful mother can keep her child out of all accidents.

Playing too much with a child will spoil him.

A parent must never make mistakes in front of the child.

Parents should sacrifice everything for their children.

When the father punishes a child for no good reason the mother should take the child's side.

A mother has to suffer much and say little.

Most children are toilet-trained by 15 months of age.

Children who take part in sex play become sex criminals when they grow up.

A child should not plan to enter any occupation that his parents don't approve of.

Too much affection will make a child a "softie."

I believe you will agree with me that the mental picture these statements provoke does not suggest a mother-child relationship involving warm affection for the child, as distinguished from a sense of responsibility and duty, or much capacity to respect the child as a separate personality with a right to his own privacy, individuality and desires.

I should not labor this point for I do not feel that child-parent relations determine schizophrenia, and there is a wide gap between typical *differences* of attitude of mothers of schizophrenics as contrasted with mothers of non-schizophrenics and typical *attitudes* of mothers of schizophrenics. We do not know, furthermore, how far these attitudes may be a result, rather than a cause, of the schizophrenic breakdown in the son. Yet we would be ignoring strong implications if we did not recognize here indication that the lack of an emotionally satisfying child-parent relationship appears to be an important factor predisposing toward a schizophrenic breakdown. Furthermore the element which is likely to be unsatisfying is not overt maternal rejection such as typically we see in the background of the unsocialized aggressive child who in extreme cases becomes the amoral psychopath, nor is it the insecure anxiety-ridden clinging to parental standards in the hope of retaining parental love and approval which typically is characteristic of the overconforming personality predisposed to psychoneurotic breakdown. Rather it is the background of the child who has learned by experience that the price of real emotional contact with the mother is the surrender of his individuality, and that even such surrender does not result in affection or in his acceptance as a person in his own right. His initial interpretation of the gentlest human approach is likely to be that it is an invitation to the surrender of individuality. And, thank you, he isn't having any.

Persons who grow up with parents who do not treat them as personalities in their own right are not easily socialized. They want and yet they fear contact with others. Their experience has been that if they begin to develop close relations with others, they do not find their feelings and desires respected, but rather that these others seek to control their behavior or even how they think and feel. Better be lonely and oneself than to lose one's individuality. The young person may turn away from others in that reaction we call schizoid withdrawal, or may timidly and halfheartedly approach them but with strong feelings of ambivalance.*

To these comments on certain tendencies to withdrawal, I would now add the observation that social withdrawal is unhealthy and sometimes precedes or leads to psychotic disorganization. Certainly it *contributes* to such disorganization, for when an individual stops checking the validity of his own observations or his own thinking against those of others, he is likely to begin to go astray. The reader may note that in the examples to follow, schizoid traits other than simple withdrawal are included.

An early effort to describe the schizoid child and his particular background occurred from a further working of material from the 500 Michigan Child Guidance Institute cases and was published with Sylvia Glickman in 1946.[26] We selected 57 cases out of the 500 for the presence of at least 3 of the 6 traits, *fantastic thinking, changes in personality, daydreaming, lack of concentration, carelessness* and *regression toward infancy.*

We stated from that study:

So far as the present study goes, it suggests factors which may contribute to the schizoid type of withdrawal. The most significant appears to be a perfectionistic mother driving toward a close, yet harsh relationship. Other factors might be interpreted to suggest a relatively good intelligence and a lack of aptitude for manual and athletic accompishment. Such a situation would create pressures and frustrations from which the child might well escape only by schizoid withdrawal into a world of fantasy. An alternative explanation which is less attractive to the authors would be that the schizoid tendency present in this group has, even at this incipient stage, reduced performance function below verbal function.

The computer clustering of the Ann Arbor material[12] revealed a cluster of children with at least three of the six entries, *seclusive, shyness or timidity, absence of close friendships, apathy, underactivity, depressed or discouraged attitude.* (While none of these traits were used in the selection of the 57 cases already reported,

---

* The above material is quoted in large part from a previous study[7] by the author, which appeared in the *Journal for Physical and Mental Rehabilitation.* Reprinted by permission.

all of these traits were significantly more frequent in the 57 cases than in the remaining cases.)

There were 61 cases so selected among 500, 21 per cent girls, and the interquartile age range was 9 to 14. While we did not have the data to determine the overlap of this material with the 57 cases selected earlier, it was doubtless very substantial.

In comparing the family background of this group with the overanxious children, the incidence of a mentally inadequate mother or of the mother handicapped by chronic illness (or serious crippling or physical impairment) was on both counts, disproportionately frequent.

In the clustering of Ackerson's cases,[25] a cluster of the schizoid child appeared both with the boys and with the girls. The central traits listed for the boys were *absentmindedness, "queerness"*—patient considered by others as mentally peculiar or crazy, *seclusiveness, listlessness, inefficiency in work or play, daydreaming* and *lack of initiative.* For the girls the central traits were *"queerness," changeable moods, depressed or discouraged attitude, question of change of personality, daydreaming, inefficiency in work or play* and *emotional instability.* Probably a cluster of clinic adolescents showing these traits would include some cases in which a diagnosis of schizophrenia could be justified. We have not excluded such cases, but since they must be in a small minority, their statistical influence cannot be great. To the extent that we use the adjective *schizoid* there is perhaps some justification for this course, since this term was introduced to characterize those who bear some similarity to the schizophrenic.

The third symptom group of Kobayashi *et al.*[30] from Japan is a cluster which combines the overanxious and the withdrawing reactions. It can be separated into an overanxious cluster and a smaller cluster of *fantastic unrealistic thinking, daydreaming, apathy, seclusiveness,* and *suspiciousness.*

A group of 120 withdrawn schizoid children was separated out from the 1,500 IJR cases.[15, 16] A few of these children probably justified the diagnosis of schizophrenia. The vast majority of them certainly would not qualify for such a diagnosis. The presence of at least 2 of 6 key entries was required for inclusion in the group.

This group included 34 (83 per cent) of 41 children whose relationship with the psychiatrist was remarkably poor because their actions appeared *psychotic or bizarre,* 25 (61 per cent) of 41 whose relationship was poor because they were *suspicious and uncommunicative,* 13 (52 per cent) of 25 classified as having a poor relationship with the psychiatrist because they were *cold, apathetic, impassive.* It included 78 (46 per cent) of 168 children for whom there was recorded *play or fantasy poorly organized,* 49 (36 per cent) of 138 children of those considered by the psychiatrist as showing *peculiar actions, delusions, obsessions, compulsions, and* 85 (23 per cent) of 369 children described by the psychiatrist as *withdrawn, seclusive, daydreaming.*

The children whom we have in our withdrawn schizoid group tend to be the younger children, those below 7 years of age. The school placement is most often *kindergarten* or *first grade,* or *not in school.* With a significant frequency the IJR examination has involved an electroencephalogram.

Difficulties in the development of speech are frequently reported in the social history, sometimes failure to develop simple sentences before three years, sometimes other difficulties.

The parental attitudes toward the patient, as judged by the social worker, do not for the most part differ from that of the parents of other clinic children significantly enough to reach statistical significance. However the mother's attitude is described as *punitive* at a significantly high level. The mother described as *overly seductive* is conspicuously rare in this group. The mother does report alcoholism and chronic illness or disability in her parental home, and consistently the social worker records that the parents are having some difficulty, such as the mother's mental health.

The psychologist obtained dull-normal IQ ratings among these children with a frequency significantly more than expected. Ratings of average and above, were less than expectancy. However, the validity of the test results was often seriously questioned by the psychologist. The psychologist frequently reported evidence of *severe emotional disturbance* or of *organic impairment or deficit.*

The attitude (interest, motivation) of the child toward the

tests was most often described as *brief, distractible, unable to focus* or *uninterested, negative,* or else *required effort to motivate.* The relationship with the psychologist was typically described as *shy, withdrawn, inhibited,* occasionally *overanimated, uninhibited* and infrequently *no notable deviation—essentially good.* The manifestation of hostility was likely to be rated either as "no evidence" or as "unable to determine." From the projective test results the psychologist typically rated the type of disturbance as *severe.* The prognosis for psychotherapy was likely to be rated as *poor.*

In the psychiatrist's ratings the primary problem area was *personality difficulties.* Among the child's problems were *destructiveness* and *retarded or progress unsatisfactory* in learning.

Aside from the personality traits on which members of this group were selected, we find them characterized as *generally immature* and *chronically anxious and fearful,* and as *depressed, discouraged* and as *noticeably depressed. Speech defect* is frequent. The child does not show a *tendency to reach out* in his relation with the psychiatrist.

Special features of the interview are *difficulty in separating from the mother, motor restlessness or incoordination.* The psychiatrist typically thought the child *severely disturbed* but did not find the *psychodynamics evident verbally or in play.*

A conspicuous (and presumably dynamic) factor in the family situation was the disproportionately frequent estimate of the mother's state as *psychosis or borderline psychosis.* Dynamic factors noted by the psychiatrist with more than usual frequency were *acquisition of new siblings or parent.* The father's reactions to the child's primary problem was frequently characterized as *indifferent, detached, minimized.* The mother's relationship with the child was frequently characterized as *overly permissive.* The mother's relationship was characterized as *infantilizing, overprotective,* not as *controlling, rigid.* Both parents' relationship was described as not *pushing to early responsibility.*

The parental relationship was characterized by *marked suspiciousness* and/or *jealousy* but by a relative absence of *marked overt sexual conflict,* and was unlikely to involve the parents' being *markedly different in background.*

In the intake information study,[28] 12 definitely withdrawn schizoid children and 10 considered questionably so, were compared with the remaining 278 cases.

The parents described these children as *seclusive* and *resentful*. They reported sleep difficulty in that the child "cannot go to sleep."

Like the brain-damaged children, these children were not accepted as equals by their peer group and were likely to be teased.

Both parents typically reported more harmony than conflict in the marital relation.

In seeking to understand these children, we might reflect that man is a social animal—but sometimes he gets tired of it! Have we not all of us, at some time or times, felt that we had had enough of the human race? Social experience is *not* always rewarding, even to those who consider themselves socialized.

Consider the lot of the social rejects, of those who do not win acceptance and do not have acceptance. If social contact frequently results in rejection, the natural protective course is to withdraw from human contact. Why risk rejection?

The big transition of childhood comes at the kindergarten and/or the first grade level. Up to this point the child has been sheltered in the family obligation toward him. The highest incidence of the *withdrawing reaction* is in the age range 5 to 7 and in those in kindergarten or first grade, or presently not in school.

Speech difficulties are more frequent in the withdrawing children than in the clinic population as a whole, and certainly speech difficulties, which make communication difficult, encourage withdrawal.

The maternal attitude seems a little less wholesome than the clinic average and seems contributory, with the mothers tending to be *critical, depreciative*. The mother from an alcoholic household, the mother with the chronic illness or disability, the mother with a mental health problem, are all disproportionately frequent in this group. This group, compared with the total clinic population, has an over-representation of children with dull and border-

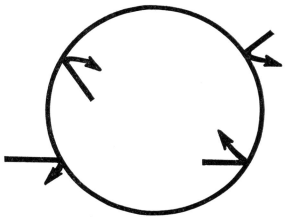

Figure 2.   Sketch of the Withdrawing Reaction.

line intelligence, and an under-representation of children of superior and very superior levels.

In such family atmosphere, is a child's withdrawal surprising?

The withdrawing reaction is another reaction which can be diagramed, as in Figure 2. An abnormally heavy protective barrier is developed around the surface of the personality. This has two effects. External stimuli often glance off and do not penetrate the protective barrier. They are not perceived. Internal impulses do not come into external actions, but are reflected autistically back into the personality.

Brad was the only child of his mother and of the second marriage of his father. Brad's father had a daughter by his first wife. This first marriage ended in divorce.

Both of Brad's parents intermittently had received psychiatric treatment. Brad's father was a salesman, not very successful, who moved a good deal and declared bankruptcy several times. He sought treatment at Mental Health Centers.

Brad's mother was a good student in school until age 13, when she began to lose interest in school and developed compulsions such as handwashing, retracing her steps, and not stepping on cracks in the sidewalk. After her marriage at the age of 23 she was very dependent on her husband and very much closed-in in the house. She too had care at a Mental Health Center and several hospitalizations.

Brad's early development was not deemed remarkable in any way. His mother did relate that because of her own emotional problems she did keep him confined and restricted. As a young child she kept him much in his play pen because it bothered her when he got into things. He never developed good sleeping patterns. He would be up much of the night and would sleep parts of the day. His adjustment to kindergarten was not considered very good. In school he was a good student and became a perfectionist. He had few friends and was often ridiculed or harassed by the other students. Outside of school his preoccupation was in earning and saving money. He worked at many part-time jobs and with the money he earned he was able to buy such things as a color television set for his family. Brad's father, meeting financial difficulties, tended more and more to borrow money from Brad. He did not pay this back, and the relation between father and son deteriorated.

When Brad was 16 both his parents were examined in a Mental Health Center. The father was seen as a person with many neurotic problems. His diagnosis was **inadequate personality.** His mother was showing obsessive-compulsive behavior and the question of a schizophrenic reaction was raised. Several months later, Brad himself was seen at the Mental Health Center. Brad was seen as anxious and apprehensive, with an incredibly bad self-image, and as one who saw himself as unable to do anything right. The admission note recorded a diagnostic impression of **adjustment reaction of adolescence,** severe, with obsessive-compulsive, depressive and schizoid features.

Brad had an extensive program of mental testing. His MMPI had suggested longstanding somatic complaints, confused thinking, aloofness, and feelings of hostility. When asked to describe himself in three words, Brad chose **indecision, lost,** and **one for perfection.**

Brad had been a capable student. He had, however, shown increasing withdrawal. He was admitted to a day hospital program at the Mental Health Center, and since he was no longer equal to attending school, his instruction was a part of the homebound program.

A year and a half later when Brad was 17 his father suffered a stroke which proved fatal. Brad's mother was hospitalized, and Brad was placed temporarily in a children's institution.

While in the children's home, Brad drank a bottle of ant poison after going to bed. In the early morning hours he became ill with influenza-like symptoms of temperature elevation, perspiration and pallor, and he began to vomit. He did not disclose that he had taken poison, nor was it suspected. In the morning he complained of stomach pains and was sent to the day hospital. Here, on interview he disclosed what he had done and was immediately sent to the general hospital where his stomach was pumped. After two days he was transferred to the psychiatric unit. From here, after 25 days, he was admitted to a state mental hospital.

Brad was offered admission to the adolescent ward. He feared that he would not be able to make an adjustment there because of his difficulties in getting along with those of his own age. At his request, accordingly, he was admitted to a men's ward. However, he was put first in school, then in other adolescent activities, and after a few days, he was moved to the adolescent ward. He tolerated this change quite well.

Brad had some idea that he wanted to become a scientist. He liked science fiction, and he had fantasies of developing a ray gun which would disintegrate mountains and make tunnels.

Reference has already been made to the obsessive-compulsive symptoms of Brad's mother. He disclosed that she would switch off the lights and switch them on again a counted number of times and ask Brad to do this with the television. Brad would refuse or would get her mixed up. "I used to think it kind of fun to make her act crazy." When asked why he did not consider his mother's feelings in this matter, his response was, "I always just think about myself. Probably that is part of my sickness."

In relation to his suicidal attempt, Brad said that he hoped to join his father in an afterlife. He also revealed that this father, in moments of discouragement, would suggest to Brad that he, the father, ought to take the boy's mother out in the car with him and get them both killed, so that Brad would have all the insurance money.

Brad spent much effort trying to persuade various members of the hospital staff to treat him by hypnosis, or to refer him to someone who would do so. This was not regarded as a constructive suggestion and consequently was not taken up. He was, however, encouraged to relax. Since he found security in the hospital and feared discharge, he became afraid of relaxing further lest he be discharged from the hospital. He also expressed some concern that he might be a latent homosexual, and this created some fear.

Presently Brad is making good progress in learning to relate to other adolescents. Although he had no confidence in his athletic ability, he proved to be a good ping-pong player. We are very hopeful about the future, for Brad has good abilities and work habits that will serve him better as an adult than as an adolescent. He is gradually gaining confidence in himself.*

Any discussion of the treatment of the withdrawing reaction will bear some relation to the ancient fable of Aesop concerning the contest between the North Wind and the Sun, as to which would succeed in making the traveler take off his cloak. The harder the North Wind blew, the more tightly the traveler wrapped his cloak about him. One cannot force a patient to give up his cloak of withdrawal. Efforts to do so will only increase his withdrawal and isolation. One can only offer him the warmth of the sun and patiently wait for his gradually loosening his defenses a little at a time, until he gains enough confidence not to need to withdraw and until he finds more satisfaction in participation than in withdrawal.

---

* Since this was written Brad left the hospital for a vocational rehabilitation program in which he did well. He is presently employed in a sheltered workshop. He has gradually improved in his capacity for social participation.

CHAPTER 12

THE HYPERKINETIC REACTION

(The "Antsy")

IN ALL OF THE REACTIONS SO FAR CONSIDERED, THE MAJOR DETER-
MINING FACTOR HAS BEEN THE RESPONSE OF THE INDIVIDUAL TO
ENVIRONMENTAL PRESSURES. WHILE UNDOUBTEDLY THERE ARE
IMPORTANT ELEMENTS OF PREDISPOSITION ENTERING INTO THE
DETERMINATION OF THESE REACTION PATTERNS, STILL THE FORE-
GOING REACTIONS APPEAR TO BE PRIMARILY A RESPONSE TO EXTERNAL
STIMULI, UNDERSTANDABLE IN TERMS OF THE FEELINGS AND RE-
ACTIONS OF HUMAN BEINGS IN GENERAL.

In the case of the *hyperkinetic reaction,* we are dealing with a
kind of reaction not equally explainable in terms of external
stimuli, but one which involves *a disposition toward over-
reactivity* on the part of the organism itself.

Jerry was 10 when he was brought to the Child Psychiatry
Service. His father was an educated man who had moved from one
academic community to another, leaving the status of a graduate
student for a faculty position. There were two boys in the family.
According to the intake application filled out by the mother, the
reasons for the referral were "poor school performance, anxieties,
and inability to get along with peers over extended periods." The
traits checked by the mother on a checklist were **impulsive,
sensitive, resentful, quick-tempered, emotional, affectionate, con-
siderate and untruthful,** the last qualified by the written word
"sometimes." As an incapacity she listed "inability to concentrate"
and as his underlying difficulties she entered, "fighting, inability
to concentrate for extended periods." The mother noted that the

111

boy did much better during the summer months when school was out. She described him as responsible, pleasant and well-behaved then but added, "during the school term his inability to concentrate hinders him enormously."

Jerry was the product of his mother's first pregnancy. The mother fell when 7½ months pregnant and then went into labor. She was taken to the hospital and delivered soon after arrival, reportedly after only 45 minutes of labor. The brith weight was 5 lbs. 10 oz. and the mother reported that there was a "dent" in his forehead at birth. Apparently there was no need for resuscitation or special measures.

Jerry's mother had had an unhappy childhood and intermittently felt insecure in her husband's affection: apparently this related more to her special needs than to any clear deficiencies in his behavior, but as a result she was an anxious and over-reactive woman. She did have some problems with the boy in toilet training. Jerry had very large hard stools. He often withheld and she resorted to enemas in toilet training.

Jerry was rather awkward, impatient in such tasks as tying his shoes but in general the development milestones seemed normal until he started school. There he was hyperactive and unable to concentrate on specific school tasks. His handwriting was poor. He had great trouble keeping friends. He had frightening dreams.

He was referred by his parents to a clinic service and was diagnosed as a neurotic child with internalized problems and a great deal of free-floating anxiety. He was seen in play therapy sessions twice a week for 14 months and his mother was seen every second week.

Jerry's mother was an anxious, sensitive woman who often over-reacted and then felt guilty about it. Jerry's younger brother seemed "the perfect child" by contrast to Jerry. Jerry was jealous of this brother because of the parental approval, and much of this came out in the play sessions.

It was the therapist's feeling that much had been accomplished when the family moved, but that therapy should be continued another year.

At the Child Psychiatry Service the problem was recognized to fit the pattern of the hyperkinetic child. Several soft neurological signs supported this impression. He could not sit still nor balance on one foot. His postural reflexes were immature. There was a shaky finger-to-nose test with past pointing of at least two inches in touching his nose with his left hand.

Psychological testing revealed at least average intelligence and a rather wide scatter. He showed an adequate visuo-motor performance.

On the basis of the clinical picture a trial of a cerebral stimulant was proposed. The parents were initially much opposed to medication, but when the school began to complain about the boy's hyperactivity and impulsiveness they agreed to a trial of methylphenidate before breakfast and lunch. This proved very successful. He ceased to be a problem in school and settled down there nicely. His handwriting improved. His nightmares ceased.

After seeing an educational film on the hyperactive child, Jerry's mother related that she remembered being particularly troubled at Jerry's unwillingness to cuddle and accept nursing, and she responded, as was described in the film, with deep discouragement and feeling of incompetence as a mother.

Jerry's teacher found that she could recognize when a dose of medication was omitted, and Jerry tended to become more of a problem for the family in the evening, when the noon dose wore off, and a smaller third dose was added in the afternoon.

Jerry's initial performance on the Iowa Test of Basic Skills was at the 13th percentile, in work study skills in the 5th grade. After he was put on methylphenidate his performance in work study skills moved up to the 52nd percentile in 6th grade and the 62nd percentile in the 7th grade.*

The foregoing illustrates an instance of the hyperkinetic reaction which was treated initially as though it were an over-anxious reaction or a neurosis. While this treatment was doubtless of some benefit, it was very time-consuming and the failure to recognize the hyperkinetic nature of the problem resulted in a failure to relieve unwarranted maternal anxiety to the extent

------

* I am indebted to Dr. Hunter Comly for this case.

that it might properly have been relieved. In those instances in which a cerebral stimulant can resolve the problem, the physician who fails to use it is not fulfilling his responsibility.

The original clustering of Ackerson's 5,000 IJR cases[1, 25] yielded just three clusters, the socialized delinquent cluster, the unsocialized aggressive cluster, and the overinhibited cluster. In going back over the clusters studied, we note that when the rules were changed so that, if the same trait appeared in two clusters, it would not be used to select further traits for either cluster, it was possible to increase these three clusters to five.

One of these clusters was called the cluster of the *brain-injured child*. In the case of the boys, the central traits were: *question of change of personality, mental status, or behavior dating from some specific event or episode; question or diagnosis of encephalitis; irritability; changeable moods; "queerness"* (defined earlier); *emotional instability; contrariness; nervousness;* and *irregular sleep habits or insomnia.* For the girls, the cluster traits were: *restlessness; question or diagnosis of encephalitis; distractibility; nervousness; violence; question of change of personality; temper tantrums; restlessness in sleep; disturbing influence in school;* and *changeable moods.*

It is noteworthy that without the additional rule stated, with both boys and girls, these two clusters flow into and disappear into, the unsocialized aggressive clusters.

It is also worthy of note that in only one per cent of the boys and one per cent of the girls is there the entry: *question or diagnosis of encephalitis.* It is of substantial interest that the period covered during which these children were examined (1923-1927) was a period in which behavioral and organic sequelae of the great epidemic of *encephalitis lethargica* were very frequent at the Institute. That is to say, *in very few of these cases could a diagnosis of encephalitis be made, or could the question even be legitimately raised on a clinical basis;* yet we are discussing a behavioral cluster such as appears when encephalitis is diagnosed or suspected.

A computer clustering[12] of behavior traits of 500 children catalogued at the Michigan Child Guidance Institute yielded five clusters. One was a hyperkinetic-distractible group of 76 cases having at least three of the six traits *hyperactive, lack of concentration, mischievousness, inability to get along with other children, overdependent,* and *boastfulness.* Only 16 per cent were girls and the typical age was 9 to 11.

The study by Kobayashi *et al.*[30] of boys judged to be problem children by psychologists in child guidance centers in Tokyo yielded a cluster with the "primary" symptoms of *lack of concentration, carelessness,* and *hyperactivity.* The "secondary" symptom was *mischievousness.* The "peripheral" symptoms were *staying out late at night, general lack of self-control, boastfulness, "weak will,"* and *unkindness.*

The facts are clear that there is an over-reactive hyperkinetic behavioral cluster which may be found strictly on the behavioral level without any reference to neurological signs or medical diagnosis. However, if one includes such neurological signs in the matrix, they relate to and become a part of the cluster.

That is to say, this group of behavioral traits forms a behavioral syndrome which is more than usually frequent in individuals who give neurological evidence of organic brain damage, but it also occurs in the great many children who do *not* clearly show such evidence.

Our 1,500 IJR cases[14, 15] included 265 in an organic-hyperkinetic cluster selected as follows.

Our organic-hyperkinetic group was selected both in terms of signs of organic brain damage and in terms of symptoms of hyperkinesis. Again, at least two of the seven criterion items were required for the inclusion of a case. The selection of 265 children in this group was based on the presence of at least two of the entries. These were *neurological impairment, organic impairment or deficit, brief-distractible-unable to focus, encephalitis or other brain damage, overanimated-uninhibited,* a history of *convulsions,* and *motor restlessness or incoordination.*

The organic hyperkinetic group included 69 (97 per cent) of 71 children who showed proven or probable signs of organic *neurological impairment.* It included 101 (87 per cent) of 116 children in whom the psychologist found symptomatic evidence of *organic impairment or deficit,* 31 (89 per cent) of 37 children in whom the social worker secured a history of *encephalitis or other brain damage,* 67 (79 per cent) of 85 children whom the psychologist rated as *overanimated-uninhibited,* and 123 (75 per cent) of 165 whose interest the psychologist rated as *brief-distractible-unable to focus.*

It also included 41 (73 per cent) of 56 children with a history of *convulsions* and 128 (54 per cent) of 237 children showing *motor restlessness or incoordination* in the psychiatric examination.

The children in the organic-hyperkinetic group are over-represented in the ages below eight and are under-represented in the ages beyond ten. This is in accord with the fact that these problems are recognizable early and, at least in the milder cases, tend toward slow improvement. As might be expected, referral is typically from a medical source.

Parental concern was probably reflected in the fact that the father as well as the mother was more likely to be involved in giving the social history than in the average clinic case. However, the father was likely to be ambivalent toward the referral and evasive or defensive about giving information. *Premature births* are frequent in this group and *easy weaning* infrequent.

A previous study of the parental response of parents of brain-damaged children[28] has indicated that delay in motor development without corresponding delay in speech or in toilet-training was most characteristic of a group. The most frequent delay was in crawling and the somewhat-less-frequent delay in walking was taken as an indication of the typical slow improvement in these children.

Delay in walking past 18 months was more than usually frequent in these IJR children and *lack of exploratory and motor freedom and courage* was highly characteristic.

Speech retardation, *no simple sentence before 3 years,* was very frequent among these children, and *present speech defect* was exceedingly common. Much of this speech defect appeared to be an articulatory difficulty and to relate to poor coordination and clumsiness of the muscles of speech. There is also some greater-than-usual frequency of *infantile speech.* The comment,

"No difficulties," in the development of speech was selectively absent.

Operations and injuries to the child were more than usually frequent. The methods of discipline used by parents did not differ from those used in other clinic cases except that *withdrawal of privileges* as a method of discipline was infrequent.

The number of instances in which the mother was not married to the father at the time of the patient's conception is significantly less than the clinic average. The social worker describes both the mother's attitude and the father's attitude toward the patient as *infantilizing, overprotective.* However, these mothers are significantly less likely than the average clinic mother to be described as either *overly seductive* or as *rigid, controlling.*

As might be expected, the psychologist obtained more intelligence test ratings of below average (including dull-normal) than with the clinic populations as a whole, and fewer ratings of average and above. There were substantially more than a proportional number called *unclassifiable* and more than an average number of *severe emotional disturbance* in this group.

The relationship with the psychologist included not only *overanimated, uninhibited* which was used in the selection, but also *provocative.* The patient's relationship with his environment was unlikely to be classified as *withdrawn, passive* and the manifestation of hostility was unlikely to be *minimal-hostility repressed,* and his relationship with his parents was unlikely to be classified as *submissive.*

The psychiatrist lists as problems of the child, *destructiveness* and *temper. School truancy, lying* and *running away from home* are less frequent than with the clinic population as a whole. *Retarded* or *progress unsatisfactory* in learning is very frequent. *Generally immature* is a personality characteristic often interfering with peer relations. Another personality characteristic which appears very prominent is *restless, excitable.* These children are unlikely to be described as *depressed, discouraged,* as *overly conforming, submissive* or as showing *fear of school* or *reluctance to attend.*

Speech defect again, as noted by the psychiatrist, is conspicuously common, and the incidence of *soiling* is significantly high.

The psychiatrist is most likely to classify the primary problem area as either *learning defects* or *somatic dysfunction*.

If the relation made by the child with the psychiatrist is essentially good, it lacks any *tendency to be reserved*.

If poor it is *overanimated, uninhibited*. If markedly poor, the child is even characterized as *psychotic or bizarre acting*.

Special features of the interview, besides *motor restlessness or incoordination,* which was used as a selective factor, are *speech defect, difficulty in separating from mother* and *play or fantasy poorly organized,* all of which showed a frequency above the clinic average.

The psychiatrist's impression was that the child was *severely disturbed*.

Both parents were thought by the psychiatrist to be over-anxious about the child. The mother was considered to be somewhat *infantilizing, overprotective* and not to be *controlling, rigid*. She was characterized as not "setting an example for the child's pathology." The father was less likely than other clinic fathers to *delegate parental responsibility to others*.

In the intake information study in Iowa City,[28] we found 22 children we believed showed definite evidence of brain damage, and an additional 27 in which we felt this evidence to be questionable. We compared these 49 cases with the remaining 251.

In these children the problem was typically noticed before the age of six.

The child was likely to be referred to the clinic by the school for school difficulty.

Parents were prone to describe these children as *spoiled*.

The child was not accepted as an equal by his peer group and was likely to be teased.

He was likely to receive special help in school.

The mother was likely to have been in poor health for the first six months after delivering this child. The parents reported the child suffered from periods of high fever.

Motor development was slow. With a disproportionate frequency, the child did not crawl before 10 months of age, did not stand alone before 13 months, did not walk alone before 16 months.

The father reported the child to be more difficult to handle them most children and, in describing the family, was likely to check "mother and father are very close to each other, but the child is not close to either."

The problems of the child with a hyperkinetic reaction in a home without effective parenting are well illustrated in the case of Phillip in Chapter 7.

It seems reasonable to presume that the hyperkinetic reaction is an expression of a delay in the functional organization of the nervous system. Most of the traits observed are those which would appear normal in a younger child—the restlessness, inability to maintain concentration, distractibility, impulsiveness. I have hypothesized that this represents a delay in the development of the dominance of the cerebral hemispheres in the control of behavior. In any event it is a fact that most hyperkinetic children show improvement on cerebral stimulants. Dextroamphetamine or methylphenidate are widely used, the latter in doses two or three times as large as the former.

We commonly give such medication two or three times daily, once on awakening or at least a half hour before breakfast, a half hour before lunch, with sometimes a third and smaller dose after school. The effect is at times so conspicuous that a teacher or parent will recognize clearly from the child's behavior when a dose has been omitted. It is best to begin with a small dose and increase it at about 5-day intervals under close contact with the family until the desired effect is obtained, an undesirable side effect becomes a problem, or until the dose is up to .1 mg/kg body weight for dextroamphetamine or .2 mg for methyphenidate. We usually drop out the dose in summer or cut it in half as hyperkinesis is better tolerated when children are not confined in school.

When children do respond to this medication, the favorable effect upon their schoolwork and their behavior is often striking.

If there is doubt about the value of such medication in a particular case, this question is easily resolved by omitting the medication for a few days while conditions are otherwise stable. The school performance and behavior are usually the most sensitive indicators.

If it is clearly of benefit, such medication should be continued until the child has outgrown the need. This typically occurs at least by the middle teens.

Common side effects are interference with sleep and interference with appetite and occasionally, symptoms of abdominal pain. Interference with night sleep rarely occurs if the medication is given early in the day. Interference with appetite in the under-weight child can be a problem. Attention to a good evening meal and a bedtime snack usually can offset this.

Although the hyperkinetic picture is the commonest one, some children suspected of minimal brain damage or dysfunction show hypokinetic symptoms and still may benefit from cerebral stimulants. Children with learning disabilities related to poor visuo-motor capacities often benefit.

We have known of no instance in which this medication led a child who needed it to the abuse of amphetamines.

CHAPTER 13

INTERRELATIONS

THE FOREGOING REACTIONS ARE, OF COURSE, NOT UNRELATED. REFERENCE ALREADY BEEN MADE TO THE FREQUENCY WITH WHICH THE HYPERKINETIC REACTION CONTRIBUTES TO THE DEVELOPMENT OF THE UNSOCIALIZED AGGRESSIVE REACTION. ACHENBACH,[3] IN PARELLEL FACTOR ANALYSES OF THE SYMPTOMS OF 300 MALE AND 300 FEMALE CHILD PSYCHIATRIC PATIENTS FOUND THE "INTERNALIZ-ING" SYMPTOMS WE HAVE CALLED "OVERANXIOUS," AND THE "EX-TERNALIZING" SYMPTOMS WE HAVE CALLED "UNSOCIALIZED AGGRES-SIVE" AT OPPOSITE ENDS OF ONE BIPOLAR FACTOR.[3] TAKING IT OUT ON THE SELF (INTROPUNITIVE) AND TAKING IT OUT ON OTHERS (EXTRAPUNITIVE) ARE ALTERNATIVE AND CONTRASTING METHODS OF REACTING TO STRESS OR DISAPPOINTMENT.

Table 1 reveals the interrelationships of the five major groups from the 1,500 IJR cases.

One point of interest is the overlap of the *organic-hyperkinetic* group with the *unsocialized aggressive* group, and particularly with the *withdrawn schizoid* group. This is interpreted to indicate that organic brain pathology and/or dysfunction contribute to both of these syndromes.

Beyond this we may note some overlap between the *over-anxious* and *withdrawn schizoid* group. These two inhibited groups have a number of characteristics in common, as was brought out in "Psychiatric Syndromes in Children and Their Relation to Family Background."[12]

Similarly, there is overlap between the *socialized delinquent* and the *unsocialized aggressive* cluster. However, the socialized delinquent relates *negatively* to the *organic-hyperkinetic* cluster.

TABLE I

PH CORRELATIONS AND P VALUES FOR RELATIONS
BETWEEN GROUPS

	Unsocialized aggressive	Socialized delinquent	Overanxious	Withdrawn schizoid	Organic-hyperkinetic
Unsocialized aggressive N=445		+.12 P<.001	−.11 P<.001	+.03 NS	+.05 P<.05
Socialized delinquent N=231	+.12 P<.001		−.01 NS	−.04 P .10	−.07 P<.01
Overanxious N=287	−.11 P<.001	−.01 NS		+.09 P<.001	.00 NS
Withdrawn schizoid N=120	−.03 NS	−.04 P<.10	+.09 P<.001		+.10 P<.001
Organic-Hyperkinetic N=265	−.05 P<.05	−.07 P<.01	.00 NS	+.10 P<.001	

These organic-hyperkinetic children evidently do not seek, or are
not accepted in, the delinquent gang.

Of interest in this relation is a study by Müller and Shamsie[34]
of adolescent girls falling in the unsocialized aggressive, socialized
delinquent and overinhibited or overanxious groups. The socialized delinquents had the most normal EEG's. The unsocialized
aggressive had a larger amount of generalized slow activity and
a greater difference between the occipital and temporal peak
frequencies. These were the most pathological records. The
overinhibited girls showed more fast activity in temporal areas, a
stronger reaction to eye-opening and more positive spikes during
chlorpromazine-induced sleep than the others. These facts are
of course in accord with the idea that organic brain damage or
dysfunction is likely to be a contributing factor to the *unsocialized
aggressive reaction,* but not to the *group delinquent reaction.*
These authors conclude: "It appears therefore that Jenkins
groups represent biological as well as psychosocial syndromes,
in which certain types of electrical brain activity indicate predispositions to certain types of behavior, and perhaps also
vulnerabilities to certain types of environmental pathology."

As might be expected, the largest negative correlation is

between the socialized delinquent and the overanxious clusters. Overanxious children are typically more inhibited than they are aggressive. And, since the gang is, to some extent at least, a security system, its members often have their level of anxiety reduced by the psychological support of their fellows and their sense of belonging.

When we consider the two entries *group stealing* and *running away from home*, both are correlated with the socialized delinquent cluster at the +.33 and +.43 levels respectively, and these correlations are significant well beyond the .001 level. This is to be expected, of course, since both of these entries were used in the selection of the socialized delinquent group. None of the other groups are significantly related to group stealing. Some of the relations are, in fact, negative, but the numbers involved are so small that the deficits do not reach statistical significance. The withdrawn schizoid group has no representatives, where 4 would be expected on a chance basis, and the overanxious groups have only 4, while 9 would be expected on a chance basis.

On the other hand, the entry *running away from home* is positively correlated with the unsocialized aggressive group ($r = +.09$, $P < .01$) and negatively correlated with the organic-hyperkinetic group ($r = -.05$, $P < .05$). The positive correlation between unsocialized aggressive behavior and running away from home is certainly not surprising, in view of the resemblances both in inner personality structure and in family background between the unsocialized aggressive child and the runaway child.

If in relation to our 1,500 IJR cases[14, 15] we seek to ask the question, *What are the differences in the quality of the parental relationships that characterize the withdrawn schizoid child, the overanxious child and the unsocialized aggressive child?* certain consistencies appear.

The mother of the withdrawn schizoid child is more likely to be rated as *psychotic or borderline psychotic;* the mothers of overanxious and unsocialized aggressive children are more likely to be rated as showing a *character disturbance or psychoneurosis* —presumably a character disturbance in the case of the unsocialized aggressive and a psychoneurosis in the case of the overanxious. It is presumably because of a greater frequency of ill-functioning mothers of withdrawn children that these mothers are likely to be non-accepting of their self-involvement in the child's problem and the fathers are more often involved in giving the history, etc. than in either of the other two groups. Also, these fathers of withdrawn, schizoid children are more frequently considered a wholesome influence on the withdrawn children than are the fathers of the unsocialized aggressive children considered a wholesome influence on their offspring. The fathers of unsocialized aggressive children are often inconsistent.

The *infantilizing, overprotective* mother is most characteristic of the overanxious child and most uncharacteristic of the unsocialized aggressive, with the schizoid falling somewhere between. However, the mothers of the schizoid children are less likely to be classified as *controlling, rigid,* than the mothers of either the overanxious or the unsocialized aggressive children. The mothers of the overanxious children are less likely to be rated as *overtly rejecting* than the mothers of either of the other two groups.

The marital relationship of the parents of withdrawn schizoid children is more likely to be affected with *marked suspiciousness and/or jealousy* than are the marriages of the other two groups.

There are differences between our groups relating to age and sex. Our hyperkinetic and withdrawing groups are younger than the other groups. Our overanxious group has a higher percentage of girls than our other groups. This fact must affect our findings and, unless we take it into account, it could result in some incorrect conclusions. Our method of connection was to pair each group with every other group and to drop out cases from both groups until the cases remaining were matched on sex and age. This of course reduced the number of significant differences by removing the sex and age differences and by reducing the size of the comparison samples. However, it does give us a set of 10 comparisons of our initial 5 groups, one with another, which are independent of age and sex. Because the comparisons have become very space-consuming to list individually, we will content ourselves with a brief characterization of important differences clearly *not* dependent on age or sex.

Summary of Characteristics

The family of the overanxious child was likely to be small, intact and with an adequate economic status. Referral was typically from a medical source. The pregnancy was *planned.* The child's relation with his environment was likely to be seen as *withdrawn, passive.* Next to the group of withdrawing children, these overanxious children were the most *withdrawn, seclusive, daydreaming.* Compared with socialized delinquents, these children were likely to prefer younger children, perhaps because compared with all but the withdrawing children, they were likely to be *victimized, teased.* They tended to be depressed and discouraged. In the psychiatric interview they were *ill at ease, apprehensive* or *passive with superficial compliance.*

Both social worker and psychiatrist saw the mothers of these children as *infantilizing, overprotective* and the psychiatrist saw them as *setting an example for the child's pathology.*

The unsocialized aggressive child is typically referred by a social agency, not a medical source. *Physical punishment* and *withdrawal of privileges* remain prominent as parental means of control. Manifestation of hostility is *excessive, easily elected.* These children are *overly competitive with siblings* and also *overly competitive with other children.* They are *restless and excitable* compared with all groups except the hyperkinetic children. The *controlling rigid* mothers and the *punitive* mothers remain prominent in the family background, presumably as important contributing factors.

The socialized delinquent tended to come from a family larger than the clinic average and, because the family was larger, to have siblings of both sexes. He was likely to be a middle child. These children came selectively from poor families, and lack of money was likely to be a cause for marital conflict. The pregnancy was usually *unplanned* and was more than usually likely to have occurred before the parents were married. Perhaps partly because of family size and space limitations, *exposure to sex activity* was more than usually frequent with these children.

Speech difficulties were unusual in these children.

As with the unsocialized aggressive child, referral is likely to be from a social agency, not from a medical source. Also, as with the unsocialized aggressive children, parental disciplinary reliance tended to be on *physical punishment* and *withdrawal of privileges*.

Lying was more prominent in these children than in any of the other groups, even though it was one of the elements used in the selection of the unsocialized aggressive groups. In *bullying, domineering, aggressive* behavior these children came next to the unsocialized aggressive group with whom it was used in selection. The problem with these children was described as *occasional* rather than *frequent or constant*. This relates to their normal behavior between delinquent episodes.

The high degree of frequency with which the fathers of withdrawing children gave the social history and actively cooperated with the clinic strongly suggests that frequently the mothers of these children are simply not adequate mothers, even though no repetitive or characteristic kind of error was demonstrated in the group.

The relation of these children to their siblings was often undetermined doubtless by reason of their poor communication.

These children were often seen as retarded in learning. *Motor restlessness or incoordination* were prominent in the psychiatrist's interview. The psychiatrist was very prone to rate these children as *severely disturbed*.

The hyperkinetic child, like the overanxious child, was likely to be referred from a medical source. The economic status of the family was adequate more often than was the case with either the socialized delinquents or the unsocialized aggressive children. The child was likely to be *restless, excitable*. *Learning defects* were frequent, as were *speech defects*. The psychiatrist was likly to see these children as *generally immature*. Compared with the socialized delinquents and the overanxious children, the play and fantasy life of these children were poorly organized.

Both father and mother were likely to be rated by the psychiatrist as reasonably wholesome. This, of course, relates to the presumption that the problems of these children have typically had an organic cause rather than one related primarily to an interpersonal basis.

Children and adolescents, even those presenting behavior problems, are human, and we can often understand other humans by putting ourselves in their shoes, psychologically speaking.

Children and adolescents often have characteristic ways of reacting to strain and adversity. If it is largely by working hard at "being good," by tightening down excessive inhibitions, we may see the *overanxious reaction* which verges toward the psychoneurotic. If it is largely by defiance and aggression, we may see the *unsocialized aggressive reaction* which verges toward the antisocial. If it is by joining with others in group rebellion, we see the *group delinquent reaction* which verges toward the criminal gang. If it is largely by flight, we see the *runaway reaction.* If it is largely by withdrawal, we see the *withdrawing reaction,* which verges toward the schizoid.

It is not difficult to identify with the individual and to "feel one's way" into each of these reactions by considering the family situation in which it is most likely to develop.

The *hyperkinetic reaction* may be understood as a result of a functional immaturity of the nervous system often occasioned by slight organic brain damage and commonly reflecting minimal brain dysfunction.

We have a better chance of modifying a characteristic maladaptive response if we understand it.

EPILOGUE

No system of classification is wholly satisfactory. The preceding chapters have presented clearly detectable clusters of cases, and the foregoing discussion endeavored to promote understanding of how these typical maladaptive patterns develop, and what may be done about them.

Not all cases are typical, and when a case does not fit a category, or fits it badly, there is reason to include the category *Other Reactions of Childhood or Adolescence* as is done in DSM-II. At best this may, over a period of time, result in the definition of other reactions worthy of special descriptions. At worst, it relieves the diagnostician of pressure to do classificatory violence to the atypical case.

Years ago I composed a bit of doggerel, as follows:

> There was a dove—no matter where:
> There was a dove that thrilled the air
> With coos miraculously fair,
> (Twas said the dove must have a soul.)

> This pigeon preened before the king
> His azure tail and crimson wing.
> His golden throat began to sing
> The promptings of his joyous soul.

> The monarch marveled as he heard.
> Quoth he, "Tis such a goodly bird
> Neglect of it were quite absurd.
> Indeed, it hath a joyous soul!

> See that my kingly word be writ:
> The royal dovecot shelter it,
> Fine grain to eat, a perch to sit,
> A priest to save its joyous soul!"

The Keeper of the Dovecot cried,
"Thy word be law! The fame abide!"
Yet he returned at eventide
    The dove that had a joyous soul.

The Keeper of the Dovecot kneeled
Before the throne, and swift unsealed
His lips. His anguished words revealed
    It would not fit a pigeonhole!

The monarch's feet slid off the stool,
He gaped, and drooled a royal drool.
"What jest is this, you surly fool,
    'It will not fit a pigeonhole?' "

The Keeper shook. His mouth was dry.
His skin was wet. His pulse was high.
" 'Tis neither jest, My Lord, nor lie.
    It will not *fit* a pigeonhole!"

The monarch stiffened as he spake.
"I've pigeonholes that never break,
Of every form, and every make.
    This bird *must* fit a pigeonhole!"

The king regained composure, then
He sent for all his wisest men,
His counselors—three score and ten.
    It would not fit a pigeonhole!

They wagged their beards with faces grave.
They bent a shoe horn, broke a stave.
They begged the bird to please behave—
    It *would* not fit a pigeonhole.

They clipped its beak and claws away.
They shore its tail so fair and gay.
They plucked its crimson wings, they say:
    The bird *must* fit a pigeonhole!

The dove was in a sorry plight
Sans beak, sans tail, sans plumage bright:
The graybeards shouted in delight,
    "It fits into a pigeonhole!"

REFERENCES

1. Ackerson, L.: *Children's Behavior Problems.* II. Relative Importance and Interrelations Among Traits. Chicago, University of Chicago Press, 1942.
2. Draper, G.; Dupertius, C. W., and Caughey, J. L., Jr.: *Human Constitution in Clinical Medicine.* New York, P. B. Hoeber, 1944.
3. Garmezy, N.: Vulnerable Adolescents: Implications Derived from Studies of an Internalizing-Externalizing Symptom Dimension, in *Psychopathology of Adolescence* (J. Zubin and A. M. Freedman, eds.). New York, Grune & Stratton, 1969.
4. Hewitt, L., and Jenkins, R. L.: *Fundamental Patterns of Maladjustment: The Dynamics of Their Origin* (Monograph). State of Illinois, Springfield (Ill.), 1946.
5. Jenkins, R. L.: Motivation and Frustration in Delinquency. *Am J Orthopsychiatry, 27*:528-537, 1957.
6. ————: Problems of Treating Delinquents. *Federal Probation, 22*:27-32, 1958.
7. ————: Behind the Catatonic Defense. *J Assoc for Physical and Mental Rehabilitation, 7*:201-204, 1953.
8. ————: *Breaking Patterns of Defeat.* Philadelphia, J. B. Lippincott, 1954.
9. ————: Delinquency as Failure and Delinquency as Attainment. Reprinted from *Illinois Twenty-sixth Annual Governor's Conference on Youth and Community Service,* 1957.
10. ————: The Psychopathic or Antisocial Personality. *J Nerv Ment Dis, 131*:318-334, 1960.
11. ————: Diagnoses, Dynamics and Treatment in Child Psychiatry. *Psychiatr Res Rep,* No. 18, Am Psychiatr Assoc., pp. 91-120, 1964.
12. ————: Psychiatric Syndromes in Children and Their Relation to Family Background. *Am J Orthopsychiatry, 36*:450-457, 1966. Reprinted (Second ed.) in *Readings in the Psychology of Adjustment* (ed. by Leon Gorlow and Walter Katkovsky), New York, McGraw-Hill, 1968.
13. ————: Delinquency and a Treatment Philosophy. In *Crime, Law, and Correction* (ed. by Ralph Slovenko). Springfield, Charles Thomas, 1966, pp. 131-145.
14. ————: The Varieties of Adolescent Behavioral Problems and Family Dynamics, *Adolescent Psychiatry* (Proceedings of a Con-

ference Held at Douglas Hospital, Montreal, Quebec, June 20, 1967). Ed. by S. J. Shamsie, Schering Corp., 1968.

15. ————: Classification of Behavior Problems of Children. *Am J Psychiatry, 125*:1032-1039, 1969. Reprinted (Second ed.) in *Readings in Human Development* (ed. by Harold W. Bernard and Wesley C. Huckins). Boston, Allyn and Bacon.

16. ————: The Varieties of Children's Behavior Problems and Family Dynamics. *Am J Psychiatry, 124*:1440-1445, 1968. Reprinted (Second ed.) in *The Child: A Book of Readings* (ed. by Jerome Seidman). New York, Holt, Rinehart and Winston, 1969, pp. 149-155.

17. ————: Typen von Verhaltensstörungen bei Kindern. *Nervenarzt, 40*:197-203, 1969.

18. ————: Behavior Disorders of Childhood. *Am Fam Physician-GP, 1*:68-73, 1970.

19. ————: Diagnostic Classification in Child Psychiatry (Editorial). *Am J Psychiatry, 127*:680-681, 1970.

20. ————: Scientific Exhibit: Behavior Disorders of Childhood. *Modern Medicine*, Feb. 8, 1971, pp. 165-171.

21. ————: The Runaway Reaction, *Am J. Psychiatry, 128*:168-173, 1971.

22. Jenkins, R. L., and Boyer, A.: Types of Delinquent Behavior and Background Factors. *Int J Soc Psychiatry, 14*:65-76, 1968.

23. Jenkins, R. L., and Blodgett, E.: Prediction of Success or Failure of Delinquent Boys from Sentence Completion. *Am J Orthopsychiatry, 30*:741-756, 1960.

24. Jenkins, R. L.; Gants, R.; Shoji, T., and Fine, E.: Interrupting the Family Cycle of Violence. *J Iowa Med Soc., 60*:85-89.

25. Jenkins, R. L., and Glickman, S.: Common Syndromes in Child Psychiatry (I. Deviant Behavior Traits; II. The Schizoid Child). *Am J Orthopsychiatry, 16*:244-261, 1946.

26. Jenkins, R. L., and Glickman, S.: Patterns of Personality Organization Among Delinquents. *Nervous Child, 6*:329-339, 1947. Reprinted in *Readings in the Psychology of Adjustment* (ed. by Leon Gorlow and Walter Katkovsky). New York, McGraw-Hill, 1968.

27. Jenkins, R. L., and Hewitt, L.: Types of Personality Structure Encountered in Child Guidance Clinics. *Am J Orthopsychiatry, 14*:84-94, 1944.

28. Jenkins, R. L.; NurEddin, E., and Shapiro, I.: Children's Behavior Syndromes and Parental Responses. *Genet. Psychol. Monogr., 74*:261-329, 1966.

29. Jenkins, R. L., and Stahle, Galen: The Runaway Reaction: A Case Study. *J Am Acad Child Psychiatry, 11*:294-313, 1972.

30. Kobayashi, S.; Mizushima, K., and Shinohara, M.: Clinical Groupings of Problem Children Based on Symptoms and Behavior. *Int J Soc Psychiatry*, 13:206-215, 1967.
31. Kretschmer, E.: *Physique and Character* (Trans. second ed.). New York, Hartcourt, 1925.
32. Lewis, H.: *Deprived Children*, London, Oxford University Press, 1954.
33. Mizushima, K., and Jenkins, R. L.: Treatment Needs Corresponding to Varieties of Delinquents. *Int J Soc Psychiatry*, 8:85-160, 1962.
34. Müller, H. F., and Shamsie, S. J.: Classification des Troubles du Comportement des Adolescents et Données Electroencephalographiques. *Can Psychiat Assoc J*, 13:363-369, 1938.
35. Quay, H. C.: Dimensions of Personality in Delinquent Boys as Inferred from the Factor Analysis of Case History Data. *Child Dev.*, 35:479-484, 1964.
36. ————: Personality Dimensions in Delinquent Males as Inferred from Factor Analysis of Behavior Ratings. *J Res Crime and Delinquency*, 1:33-37, 1964.
37. Reckless, W. C.: The Etiology of Delinquent and Criminal Behavior. *Soc Sci Res Council Bull*, No. 50, 1943.
38. Rheingold, H. L.: The Modification of Social Responsiveness in Institutional Babies. *Monogr Soc Res Child Dev*, 21: No. 21-48, 1956.
39. Robins, L. N., and O'Neal, P.: The Adult Prognosis for Runaway Children. *Am J Orthopsychiatry*, 29:752-761, 1959.
40. Shaw, C.: *The Jackroller*. Chicago, University of Chicago Press, 1938.
41. ————: *Brothers in Crime*. Chicago, University of Chicago Press, 1938.
42. Sheldon, W. H.: *The Varieties of Human Physique* (Third ed.), New York, Harper & Bros., 1945.
43. Shinohara, M., and Jenkins, R. L.: MMPI Study of Three Types of Delinquents. *J Clin Psychol*, 23:156-163, 1967.
44. Szasz, T.: *The Myth of Mental Illness*, New York, Hoeber-Harper, 1961.
45. Tsubouchi, K., and Jenkins, R. L.: Three Types of Delinquents: Their Performance on MMPI and PCR. *J Clin Psychol*, 25:353-358, 1969.
46. Thomas, A.; Chess, S.; Birch, H. G.; Hertzig, M. E., and Korn, S.: *Behavioral Individuality in Early Childhood*. New York, New York University Press, 1963.
47. ————: *Temperament and Behavior Disorders in Children*. New York, New York University Press, 1968.
48. Topping, R.: The Treatment of the Pseudosocial Boy. *Am J Ortho psychiatry*, 13:353-360, 1943.

INDEX

Mother critical, depreciative, 17, 67, 68, 106
Mother, death of, 47
Mother delegating parental responsibility to others, 68, 75, 84
Mother delinquent or promiscuous, 33, **76, 95**
Mother, difficulty in separating from, 54, 60, 105, 118
Mother inconsistent, 56, 67, 68
Mother indifferent, detached, 76
Mother infantilizing, overprotective, 55, 56, 68, 75, 76, 105, 117, 118, 124, **125**
Mother overly ambitious, 68
Mother overly permissive, 68, 81, 84, 105
Mother overly seductive, 104, 117
Mother perfectionistic, 102
Mother psychoneurotic, 17, 69, 123, 124
Mother psychotic or borderline psychotic, 105, 123
Mother punitive, 67, 68, 75, 76, 104, 125
Mother pushing child to early responsibility, 105
Mother rejecting, 34-35, 37, 65, 67, 68, 75, 76, 84, 94, 101, 124
Mother rigid, controlling, 117
Mother rivalrous with child, 68
Mother setting example for child's pathology, 56, 118, 125
Mother showing marked preference for other sibling, 75, 78
Mother violent-tempered, 33
Mother working, 73
Müller, H. F., 57, 122
Murder, 32

Nail-biting, 29, 56
National Institute of Mental Health, 23
Negativism, contrariness, 65, 114
Nervousness, 53, 114
Neurological impairment, 115
Neurosis, neuroses, *see* Psychoneurosis
Negro children, *see* Black children

Negro, American Negro Community, 38
Neurotic, neuroticism, neurotic traits, *see* Psychoneurosis
New York State Training School for Boys, Warwick, 79, 80-85
Nightmares, terror dreams, 29, 54, 60, 112
Nor-adrenalin, 5
Nosology, 21

Obedient, 57
Obscene and profane language, 33, 62-63, 65
Obsessive-compulsive behavior, 108, 109
Obsessive-compulsive personality, 26
Oedipus complex, 40
Only child, 92
Organic brain syndrome, 24, 127
Organic impairment or deficit, 76, 104, 115
Organic-hyperkinetic group, 16, 115, 116, 121-127
Out-group, 30
Overanxious reaction, 16, 49-58, 103, 113, 121-127
Overdependent, 115
Overinhibited, 15, 16, 29-32, 37, 38-40, 41-42, 53, 58, 114
Overinterest in opposite sex, 73
Overinterest in sex, 33
Overly competitive, 68, 78, 125
Overly conforming, 54, 76, 101, 117
Overprotection, 31, 54, 62
Overrestriction, 31

Paranoid personality, 26
Parental, *see* Parents
Parental conflict, *see* Marital conflict
Parental disharmony, *see* Marital maladjustment
Parent-Child Relations Questionnaire, 85, 93
Parents, abusive, 36
Parents, alcoholic, 36